Palliative Care:
A Practical Guide for the Health Professional

Dedication

I would like to dedicate this book to Harry, my father, who taught me the importance of listening to other people, of walking beside them when they need companionship and of letting them go when they are ready to follow their own path.

Kathryn Boog

I wish to dedicate this book to my father, Ron Lane, for the courage, determination, love and humour he continues to show.

Claire Tester

For Elsevier:

Commissioning Editor: **Dinah Thom**
Development Editor: **Catherine Jackson**
Project Manager: **Elouise Ball**
Designer: **Charlotte Murray**
Illustrations Buyer: **Gillian Richards**
Illustrator: **Barking Dog Art**

Illustrations for chapter headings developed from Claire Tester's designs.

Palliative Care: A Practical Guide for the Health Professional

Finding meaning and purpose in life and death

Kathryn M. Boog BScOT HPCReg

Clinical Specialist Occupational Therapist in Palliative Care,
St Columba's Hospice, Edinburgh, UK

Claire Y. Tester DipCOT HPCReg

Lead Allied Health Professions Consultant Occupational Therapist in Cancer, Cancer Strategies
Team, Health Department, Scottish Executive, Edinburgh, UK

Foreword by Harvey Max Chochinov OM FRSC
Canada Research Chair in Palliative Care Director, Manitoba Palliative Care
Research Unit Professor

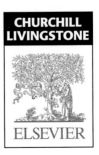

CHURCHILL LIVINGSTONE

ELSEVIER

EDINBURGH   LONDON   NEW YORK   OXFORD   PHILADELPHIA   ST LOUIS   SYDNEY   TORONTO   2008

2/1/08

Contents

SECTION 1
Exploring the impact of dying and death   1

V

Contents

VI

SECTION 3

How to survive as staff 171

Foreword

About six months ago I was contacted by Kathryn Boog and Claire Tester with a request to write the foreword for their book *Palliative Care: A Practical Guide for the Health Professional.* I am embarrassed to admit that while they knew of my own work I was unfamiliar with theirs. But something about the description of what they were attempting to accomplish with this book seemed intriguing, both in terms of scope and imagination. They used words like 'lateral thinking', 'creativity' and 're-evaluating practice'; and then there was the book's subtitle *'Finding meaning and purpose in life and death'*. All this is to say that I agreed to their request and am sincerely grateful for having done so.

There is something unique about the feeling of spending time with people who have a deep wisdom about the challenges and needs facing those confronting a terminal illness. Reading this book imparts that feeling. Kathryn Boog and Claire Tester are occupational therapists with years of experience working in an adult and children's hospice respectively. Those who assume that occupational therapy offers a narrow perspective on palliative care will find themselves pleasantly surprised. In fact, it is the solution-oriented stance that one associates with occupational therapy that makes this book both practical and extraordinarily rich. Where else might one find clinical pearls ranging from providing cutlery and pen grips to enhance a sense of regaining control, to in-depth descriptions on how to guide patients towards meaning, making generativity activities still within the patient's grasp as their condition deteriorates towards death?

While many of the challenges facing dying patients are of an existential nature, Boog and Tester remind us that angst sometimes yields to very practical solutions. In that regard they offer many suggestions whose application they have refined over many years of practice. The text is richly illustrated with numerous examples of situations and outcomes, encouraging lateral thinking and a creative approach; for example, encouraging the writing of reconciliatory letters, or expressions of love; helping a dying successful playwright create a collage – consisting of theatre reviews and personal photographs with the 'rich and the famous' – reminding her and others of her prior days of glory. While my own research on dignity has empirically examined the importance of understanding how patients perceive themselves to be seen, these two skilled and sensitive clinicians have woven these ideas into a creative approach to palliative, end-of-life care.

This book encompasses the social, psychological, emotional and spiritual influences that affect people's perceptions of their lives in relation to their actions past, present and future. It considers problems encountered on a day-to-day basis, offering clear, workable guidance and demonstrating practical solutions, based on proven theory and experience. Although practical, this book is not atheoretical, with suggestions and approaches placed within the context of a rich and diverse literature, including developmental psychology, existential philosophy, thanatology and empirical contemporary palliative care research. *Palliative Care: A Practical Guide for the Health Professional* is also unique in that it spans across the age spectrum in palliative care, including babies, small children, young adults, and adults and older people who all have life-limiting conditions.

Contemporary palliative care is often stymied in the face of existential, spiritual and psychological angst that can accompany patients nearing death. Boog and Tester challenge professionals to reconceptualise their practice by offering insights into different and creative ways of approaching given situations, based on approaches that have been used successfully by the authors, as reflected by the responses from patients, relatives and friends, and feedback from the multidisciplinary team. Although written by occupational therapists, many other professional groups will identify with the dilemmas and solutions described, not only those working in palliative care but also in the wider fields of care of the elderly and chronic illness. Instances where suggestions can be applied are often limited by the creativity of the caregiver and the lateral thinking required to implement new ideas. Dying is a unique experience that sometimes offers people the opportunity to review their lives, seek out what really matters and find peace. This book offers suggestions as to how they can be supported in that quest.

I now understand – given the nature of my own research on palliative care and interest in human dignity at the end of life – why these authors might have sought me out for the singular honour of introducing this fine and unique book. I can now say that any feelings of admiration and respect are, indeed, mutual.

Harvey Max Chochinov

Preface

For what matters above all is the attitude we take toward suffering, the attitude in which we take our suffering upon ourselves.

Viktor Frankl
(1978) *Man's Search for Meaning.* Hodder and Stoughton, London, p. 114

Palliative care is a developing field of practice which is growing as the population lives longer with long-term conditions, a higher incidence of cancer, and complex needs in co-morbidity of conditions. Many health professionals working in palliative care are lone practitioners, which will continue as care in the community continues to be developed. The practitioners working in hospices and palliative care are often pioneering new ways of working as there is little evidence-based practice as a resource. As occupational therapists the authors Kathryn and Claire, each working at an adult and a children's hospice respectively for a number of years, have been keen to develop and share their own practice and experience with health professional colleagues from different disciplines.

In palliative care the need to determine a sense of meaning and purpose in life is significant. If one considers life as meaningless and empty of purpose or reason this can be depressing and lead to a sense of regret and overwhelming sadness. Finding meaning and purpose in one's life may only be considered towards the end of that life, whenever that is. This involves thinking of achievements, of relationships, of love shared, and of things left undone. For some there is a sense of becoming a burden at the end of their life and of guilt, and depression. A readjustment to the acceptance of being terminally ill has to occur before people can begin to reflect and make sense of their life. This is a painful experience. For some patients it can be isolating as no one wants to speak of death and dying. The need to address one's actions and relationships through life, and to be at peace with oneself appear to be paramount at the end of life. What matters to the person at core through life, matters at death. For children and young adults there are varying degrees of understanding of events occurring around them, and their emotional experience must be considered. Health professionals working in palliative care have an important role here to support the patient, whatever age, and the family.

Claire's comments:

Having worked with children who had life-limiting conditions in different settings since 1983, it was when I began working at a national children's hospice 7 years ago that I realised I needed to learn more about palliative care for children. I was acutely aware of the sensitivities of children and young people who knew they had life-limiting conditions but acted out different behaviours and emotions rather than discuss or share their thoughts and feelings. By contrast parents acted cheerfully around their son or daughter but would otherwise be despairing and frightened themselves. This was at times baffling. I studied for a postgraduate diploma in Therapeutic Skills with Children and Young People at the Institute of Child Psychotherapy. What I learnt about emotional development and behaviour, different theories and approaches, the unconscious as well as institutional dynamics informed my approach. I was helped to understand and recognise behaviours and feelings of others, and my own. This was at times very upsetting as it was emotional pain I was witnessing and developing a sensitivity to, but it was this degree of sensitivity which enabled me to listen and to talk to children and young people, as well as siblings and parents, and to provide support appropriately.

From my experience and meeting other therapists, I have found that working with patients who are terminally ill and dying can often make a therapist feel deskilled, questioning one's own effectiveness. In addition the cumulative emotional effect takes its toll and it can be difficult to keep going. Some strategies I have developed are included here to support the therapist and health professional. It is my intention to share something of what I have learnt so that it may inform and support both the professional and the patient.

Kathryn's comments:

As life reaches its end, people begin to reflect on who they are, where they have come from and how they got to this place. Once their symptoms are addressed and they feel more comfortable, they may have a sense of urgency to settle unfinished business, resolve old conflicts and effect emotional closure. I have had 18 years' experience of hospice work, working from a biopsychosocial perspective, dealing with lifestyle management issues and using creative activity as a therapeutic medium to address these alongside the psychological, social, emotional and spiritual issues that influence quality of life for these patients. Despite using a creative approach for all of this time, I am still amazed at the effect such a style of intervention has on the patients' lifestyle, and in facilitating communication between them and those around them at a time when communication can be difficult. The symbolic relevance of creative activity has proved a very useful tool for both needs assessment and treatment strategy, based on core skills and coupled with lateral thinking and an imaginative approach. My own enthusiasm for this approach has been matched in recent years by the number of requests from people from both inside and outside my own profession who are keen to adopt this approach and who request information, talks and visits to learn the processes for themselves. But most of all, the hope for this book is that by using its content to direct and perfect a different style of intervention, people involved with others who are dying might begin to see them for the real, living people that they are, who want to live until they die.

In this book we have developed core occupational therapy skills, adapting and enhancing them by the use of personal life skills and lateral thinking to provide a style of therapy that can be used in a variety of settings where people begin to create the last chapter of their lives.

Edinburgh 2008

Kathryn Boog
Claire Tester

Acknowledgements

We would like to thank family, friends and colleagues for their interest and support in our work, without whose encouragement this book would not have been written.

Claire wishes to thank:

Janis Sharp for her sterling work in deciphering notes for the talk which formed the basis of the chapter 'Keeping going'.

Angus and Hamish for their generous use of the PC and their tolerance.

And especial thanks to Gordon, for his total and unswerving support, patience and understanding throughout. Thank you, I could not have done it without you.

Kathryn wishes to thank:

Robin, David, Amy and Katie for their technical and domestic support and their total confidence that I could do this.

My mother Edith, for patiently listening to my rambles, good and bad, throughout the whole process.

And last but by no means least Rosie, who took me for long doggy walks to clear my head and kept me company late into the night.

My sincere thanks to all of you. My family.

Kathryn and Claire would like to thank Dinah Thom, Catherine Jackson, Elouise Ball and all at Elsevier who have helped us so much with this book, and for their professionalism throughout.

Introduction

Palliative care is defined as 'an approach that improves the quality of life of patients and their families facing the problems associated with life-threatening illness, through the prevention and relief of suffering by means of early identification and impeccable assessment and treatment of pain and other problems, physical, psychosocial and spiritual' (WHO 2005).

Death is still a taboo subject in this liberated modern society. The people who are dying often have difficulty discussing the experience, whilst those around them may shy away or choose to ignore what is happening. People feel the need to review their lives, to finish things off, to deal with issues that have been simmering beneath the surface for years and now suddenly are pushed to the fore. They must make preparations to take their leave, to make their farewells – but how to do this? There is no best way to say goodbye. For many, it will involve seeking meaning in life, mortality and death, making and maintaining connections with others or reinstating lost relationships (Prochnau et al 2003), and so for health professionals working with patients at the end of their lives, these factors need to be considered alongside the patients' clinical needs. This will be a new viewpoint for many, and the question often is 'Where to start?'

Geoff Norman (2003) suggests that in order to become an expert, clinicians need to marry their academic and theoretical knowledge with their practical experiences gained over a period of time. By using this process, practitioners can draw on the variety of solutions that they have encountered to guide their practice, adapting and developing their approach to encompass the wide variety of needs of their patients, including those with mental health problems, learning and cognitive difficulties and the many other problems which can make this patient group complex and challenging to work with.

This book offers a presentation of theoretical and empirical evidence available, using literature from other areas of care as guidance, e.g. mental health and care of the elderly, and adopting and adapting approaches to inform and direct practice in this ever-expanding field.

This information will be developed, using stories to reflect the importance of narrative, emphasising the role of storytelling in creating a holistic picture of the person and in understanding the wider impact of the illness on the person's situation; for example, the relationship between symptoms, feelings and ability to function. Narrative and sharing stories with patients can also help transcend differences (between professions, or different cultures, for example) and facilitate communication with these others (Mattingly 1991).

The book offers new slants on old ideas, and describes new ideas that have been used successfully by the authors, as reflected by the responses from patients, their relatives and friends, and feedback from the multidisciplinary team.

Patients requiring palliative care are found in a variety of settings, and presenting with a wide variety of conditions, including cancer. People will have very different needs, depending on the stage of their illness and their personal circumstances, and the complexity of their situation may mean that health professionals feel disempowered, but this book hopes to confirm that by reflecting on past practice and adapting it for use in palliative care, and using personal life experience to extend those skills, those working with patients with life-limiting conditions will gain confidence through their experiences. By re-evaluating practice, and thinking in a different way, workable solutions can be found to empower health professionals when faced with clients with deteriorating abilities and conditions. The skills learned can then be implemented in a wide variety of settings – care of the elderly, care homes, chronic sick situations, at home, with children, for children, etc. and adapted as the need arises.

The experience of working in palliative care can be one of a personal voyage of discovery, bringing with it an acknowledgement of the complexity of human existence and a realisation of the finiteness of life, the whole process sustained by the reassurance that the opportunity for change and development can continue until the last moment, allowing people to live until they die.

References

Mattingly C 1991 The narrative nature of clinical reasoning. American Journal of Occupational Therapy 45(11):998–1005

Norman G 2003 The role of experience in the development of clinical reasoning. Editorial. International Journal of Therapy and Rehabilitation 10(11):488

Prochnau C, Liu L, Bowman J 2003 Personal--professional connections in palliative care occupational therapy. American Journal of Occupational Therapy 57(2):196–204

World Health Organization 2005 Definition of palliative care. Online. Available: http://www.who.int/cancer/palliative/definition/en/

Section 1

Exploring the impact of dying and death

Challenges in palliative care

Kathryn Boog

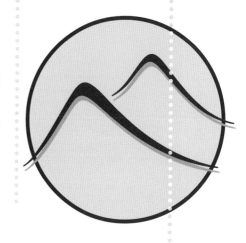

Life's challenges are not supposed to paralyse you, they're supposed to help you to discover who you are.

Bernice Johnson Reagon

Key words

evidence-based practice; establishing the role; complexity of care; core skills; palliative rehabilitation

1

Palliative care is still regarded as an emerging specialty, less than 40 years having passed since Dame Cecily Saunders founded St Christopher's Hospice, offering inpatient facilities to the dying. Over recent years, development in this area has been rapid, and now includes a wide variety of methods for the delivery of care to that patient group, adding care at home, day care, palliative interventions in acute units and care of the elderly, amongst others, to the original inpatient provision. Whilst cancer patients remain the largest group receiving palliative interventions, it is becoming increasingly recognised that people suffering from chronic, progressive illnesses, which will eventually become terminal, will require the same type of end-of-life care. Neurological conditions such as motor neuron disease and Parkinson's disease, dementia, diseases related to organ failure such as cardiac and renal conditions and chronic obstructive pulmonary disease (COPD), and many other chronic and acute illnesses would all benefit from this type of input at the appropriate stage (WHO 2004a,b). The literature also reflects the growing recognition of end-of-life requirements of care home residents (Watson et al 2006), highlighting an increasing awareness of the wide spectrum of need for palliative care in the general population and resulting in a desire for education, by health professionals, in order that they can feel equipped to offer appropriate interventions to their client group.

The needs of the dying can be complex, influenced by a wide variety of issues, and since each individual's experience will be subjective and unique, the difficulty for those interacting with people who are terminally ill can simply be knowing where to start. What is it that people most want to achieve with their restricted time; what matters to them most – and why? What skills do we already have that we can adapt to use in supporting and empowering patients on their journey through the last chapter of their life?

The needs of those caring for the dying, including the health professional, must also be taken into account, and education and learning how to adapt, and the need to learn new skills, have been identified in several publications (Allied Health Professions Palliative Care Project Team 2004, NICE 2004).

Most of the literature to date has been descriptive – qualitative studies involving small numbers of participants. This information has been used as a foundation on which the building blocks of practice development have been constructed, relating it to core skills and past and present experiences, and enabling the professional to assess the appropriateness of particular interventions. The lack of robust research studies has meant that practice must be informed by other means. Expert opinion, clinical experience and the perspectives of service users and carers can all provide an evidence base (NHS Scotland 2004), so assimilating this available information and using it to develop professionally, relating it to guidelines for practice as they become available, may well be a more relevant consideration.

The nature of a person's dying and death is shaped by numerous influences, any or all of which may require revisiting in order that the individual may be directed towards a good quality of life in the period before death. Using biography as a therapeutic way to discovering meaning is one way of achieving this (Lichter et al 1993).

Life narratives, describing roles, relationships, previous illness, hopes, dreams, cultural and spiritual issues, will all have their part to play in how the final act of that person's life is played. People may have a complex history of multiple pathologies or have underlying problems unrelated to their terminal illness, such as mental health issues, cognitive impairment, sensory deficits or communication issues, which also need to be taken into consideration.

Symptoms

Symptoms may be related to treatments and involve concerns about body image, fatigue, nausea, pain and discomfort, or they may be a means of expressing fear of dying and death. Whilst the complexities and dilemmas associated with illness are not the sole prerogative of the dying, palliative care has the added element of shortness of time in which to deal with these issues, and this is what thrusts the situation into sharp perspective.

Symptoms can be complex to control, due to a variety of underlying issues, and management of these symptoms needs to be effective for improved quality of life – the key aim in palliative care. Many patients find it easier to focus on the physical aspect of their illness, rather than acknowledge the other painful issues that are affecting their well-being, and may consciously or unconsciously avoid thinking about them, making symptom management difficult.

Psychological state, social and cultural background, environment and life experiences all influence the perceived intensity of symptoms. For example, studies indicate that there is a significant correlation not only between anxiety and dyspnoea, but also between fatigue and breathlessness (Bruera et al 2000, Tanaka et al 2002). Further, it is suggested that since breathless patients may have difficulty controlling their breathing and learning relaxing techniques because of anxiety, utilising these coping strategies for pain management may be compromised, indicating that the experience of breathlessness is one that involves elements that are unconnected to mechanical function alone (Tanaka et al 2002). Conversely, the limitations imposed by dyspnoea may be the cause of an individual's anxiety (Corner et al 1996), as can the influence of pain or fatigue.

Palliative care delivery encapsulates the notion of total pain, which again reflects the complexity of symptoms in this field (SIGN 2000). The physical restrictions imposed by the disease can be exacerbated by the emotional upheaval triggered by the diagnosis, and the resulting emotional and spiritual pain can make treatment of symptoms difficult, as the pain may manifest itself in a physical way, the patient either choosing to deny the psychological influences, or employing tactics in order to avoid confronting painful issues, such as sadness, fear, anger and multiple losses. To further complicate the issue, these emotions are often not seen by the patient as causing or influencing symptoms (Lichter 1991).

Silence is often used to hide emotional anguish and responding to pain of this nature will depend on determining and understanding its nuances. People may feel that if they do not disclose particular details about themselves, they may be liked and respected more by others, including staff and fellow patients. They now have more time on their hands, as they no longer fulfil previous roles, and they may spend this time ruminating over past fears, guilt or frustrations. Lack of energy will not only result in inability to perform certain tasks, but will also affect concentration, making it difficult for people to think clearly and logically, thereby adding to their anxieties and influencing their perception of their situation.

The individual's illness experience, then, is subjective – affected by a wide variety of internal and external factors, and therefore a person's own assessment of particular symptoms is the only true picture available to us (Bruera et al 2000).

Relationships

The end of life offers opportunities for personal growth and, for some, the deepening of relationships, but for others, it can widen the chasm between people (de Hennezel 1997). The whole family is affected by the illness process and relationships take on a greater significance for the dying person. Knowing that time is limited can, however, have the advantage of allowing time for the opportunity to revisit past pleasures once more, something denied to those who die suddenly. There can also be time for reconciliation, to say thank you, to leave legacies, or make final arrangements – in other words, to deal with unfinished business, and bring life to a satisfactory conclusion.

However, relationships can be fraught during this period for a number of reasons. Carers may not want to take on the roles that can no longer be fulfilled by the ill person. Loss of roles and losing control are major concerns for many people. For some, 'letting go' will occur earlier than for others, some of whom will need to maintain their role and feel in control right to the end in order to complete certain life tasks. They have fears of having to relinquish or change certain of these roles, seeing this as a threat to their personhood and some people may strive to maintain their influence even after death.

Patients can be angry at their situation and the people around them, and it is very difficult for loved ones to be constantly on the receiving end of this projected anger. Realising that the anger is really at the disease and loss of control over their life and their future, patients will feel guilty for the hurt they have caused and this may be further exacerbated by the inability to communicate, resulting in frustration and distress (Cassidy 1991).

People may also express a variety of feelings related to religion and existential issues, questioning personal values, and the meaning of their lives: What have I done to deserve this? Why me?

They may have concerns related to collusion and lack of trust in both personal and professional relationships, where they may test staff and relatives in order to compare information they have been given.

Modern-day advances in medicine have prolonged the period where people are living whilst dying. Families prepare themselves for the death of their loved one, only for the patient to recover unexpectedly. This living with uncertainty during many periods of relapses and remissions will put a strain on relationships, and for those that are already tenuous, the pressures can be enormous. Long-term disruption of family life and an extended period of anticipatory grief may result in the patient feeling abandoned, whilst progressive dependence on others can create feelings of becoming a burden to the family.

People have anxieties about how their death will affect others. Dying parents worry about telling the children – how much to tell them; what, when and who will do the telling. How will they cope with the separation from their child if that child cannot visit every day? What will the children's memories be of their parent? These fears are relevant in respect of adult children as well as younger ones, and will also affect relationships between dying adult children and their parents, as well as the extended family, including grandparents.

Having to carry the burden of others' fears and anxieties concerning the illness and its outcome can be exhausting emotionally for patients, as can having to deal with people who refuse to discuss the situation. Avoidance tactics may range from family and friends choosing to visit but not mention the illness, to steering clear of any contact at all. In contrast, some people may feel smothered by all of the attention that they receive, just wishing to maintain some of their previous life roles and be treated as if nothing had happened.

When people are faced with their own vulnerability, and the realisation that they are not immortal, their sense of security and well-being is challenged. Patients faced with increasing losses, such as any of their roles; physical function, including power and strength; mental ability; ability to communicate effectively; body image and independence, will consider their self-esteem and feelings of security to be threatened (Cassidy 1991, Lloyd 1989), and the loss of status and social role may result in physical and emotional withdrawal, leading to social death (Lloyd 1989). Their perception may be that, with the loss of their future, and their hopes and dreams, they see the situation as out of their control and they may begin to grieve for these losses.

6

Goals

With the acceptance of imminent death, perspectives shift and change as the important issues – what really matters – appear to become more obvious as life and time diminish. The deterioration in the clinical condition will affect the focus of goals, reflecting changing outlooks and priorities that tend towards 'getting things in order'. This may involve practical activities such as bringing certain matters to their conclusion – tying up financial or legal issues, e.g. making a will, planning the funeral or making arrangements for the care of pets – or it could relate to emotional issues, such as reconciliation, last gifts, writing cards and letters and saying goodbye, or to generativity and legacy – making memory albums and boxes. Whichever activities are chosen, they will generally involve the sorting out and rounding off of particular areas of people's lives, in order that they can reach practical and emotional closure and a state of being at peace with themselves (Lichter 1991).

Healthcare professionals

These unique challenges to the patient's sense of well-being and fulfilment are also reflected in the professionals' experience of the situation. Feelings about limited life expectancy and deterioration, relationships, coping mechanisms, keeping going, finding meaning and purpose in life and death, maintenance of dignity and feeling worthy of respect are common areas of concern. Lack of time in which to achieve desired goals is also a hurdle common to both. Exposing oneself to another human being's raw emotions, opening Pandora's box, and sharing something of oneself in the therapeutic relationship can be a new and daunting situation to contemplate. Professionals may have difficulties with being constantly exposed to painful emotional issues, and use defence tactics such as involvement in activity in order to avoid listening to or addressing these (Mackenzie & Beecraft 2004).

Several studies highlighting the needs of the healthcare professional working in palliative care indicate that best practice involves an intermingling of core skills, past experience, and reflecting on personal values and concerns (Bye 1998, Dawson & Barker 1995, Rahman 2000). Reflection is a useful measure for the development of professional practice, encouraging analytical thinking (Andrews 2000) about why and how therapeutic interventions were used (Creek 2003). It can be a way of expressing and exploring the emotions involved for the professional (Prochnau et al 2003), particularly through diary keeping, and the outcome will indicate areas where changes can be made, thereby influencing future practice.

Many professionals are building new roles involving clinical and administrative issues that are influenced not only by individuals' experience and viewpoint, but also reflect their personality and life experience, ensuring that the new role is one that they feel comfortable with. They may be lone workers in their professional group, where having to deal with role negotiation, particularly if it is a newly created post, can be a difficult task. The available literature, including studies and guidelines, can be supportive if it is used to emphasise how specific interventions can meet the criteria, in order to direct employers towards a different way of thinking. Discussion with a supervisor, and using peer support from members of a special interest group will ensure that practice is kept relevant to the particular profession, as growing experience and confidence lead to developments in the service. Active promotion of the role by educating others, for example at multidisciplinary training sessions, journal club presentations, or being involved in the orientation programmes of new staff, are ways to engender support from the multidisciplinary team and increase referrals (Rahman 2000). Carrying out joint interventions, acknowledging the grey areas of work, identifying gaps in the service and sharing the solutions with members of the team, and involvement in research and audit groups, will also highlight the role and help to consolidate it.

Professionals should feel able to admit when they have no answer to a particular problem (Lugton 2002), but should also seek help in order that the issue is addressed. Multidisciplinary teamwork is the basis of providing holistic care for the palliative care patient and members of the team are highly interdependent (Dawson & Barker 1995). Thus the importance of mutual understanding and appreciation of roles is paramount to the well-being of this patient group.

The scope for professionals working in palliative care is wide and varied, but financial constraints and pressure to comply with the model of care adopted by the institution, and colleagues' perception of what 'normal' practice should be, can be barriers to the creative approach. There may be some discord amongst professionals as to the suitability of particular interventions. The decisions not to introduce, or to discontinue, certain activities are also areas of conflict. This situation can be addressed by discussing the reasoning behind the decision, basing it on core skills, evidence – based on practice and experience – and explaining that activity can be just as effective when patients are allowed just to 'be' themselves, instead of constantly 'doing' (Needham & Newbury 2004).

Patient information leaflets, outlining the service for consumers, will also help to educate others about the role.

Professionals need to be flexible and adaptable whilst still remaining true to their professional philosophy. The approach should enable and empower the patient, revealing opportunities for progress, but yet it cannot be prescriptive, as each person and set of circumstances is unique. For this reason, it is important to take a holistic view of the situation, to find out who each person really is, and what that person really wants.

In the face of dying and death, where clients have deteriorating abilities, professionals can feel deskilled themselves, inadequate and uncertain. The need to be creative, and think laterally, not literally, is paramount in the interpretation of accumulated information and the subsequent implementation of interventions. When new ideas are introduced into the practice situation, health professionals can experience some difficulties as others within the team adjust to the different perspective taken, and may find this unsettling and challenging. Consolidation of the role by reflecting back to basic core skills and professional philosophies, directed and supported by guidelines and standards of practice for palliative care, will underpin practice and instil confidence in the practitioner.

Core skills

For occupational therapists, the core skills are defined as (Creek 2003):

1. Collaboration with the client
2. Assessment
3. Enablement
4. Problem solving
5. Using activity as a therapeutic tool
6. Group work
7. Environmental adaptation.

Collaboration with the client

Client-centred care will stem from an understanding of what is important to that person at this particular moment in time. Listening to people's personal narratives, and finding out about lifestyles, relationships, hopes and priorities, will provide very useful background information for finding out who they really are and what matters most (Carter et al 2004).

Several studies indicate that listening to someone's life story shows regard for individual dignity through the affirmation of the unique qualities and attributes of that person (Chochinov et al 2005, Kissane et al 2001). Understanding hopelessness, loss of meaning and existential distress – all recognised as the core features of demoralisation syndrome in palliative care (Kissane et al 2001) – and regaining control of a person's situation (Carter et al 2004) are recognised approaches for the preservation of dignity in the dying. Revealing more about that person's history can nurture a deeper understanding of past actions and related present concerns, and may be stimulated by the sharing of stories, albeit on a superficial level on the professional's part.

Limited self-disclosure to encourage patients to reciprocate with stories of their own will ensure that the process is singularly for the patient's benefit (Nowak & Wandel 1998), providing information relevant to that person's care. It can create the opportunity for the enhancement of the therapeutic relationship and the development of empathy and trust, the prerequisites to successful outcomes from both the professional's and patient's perspective.

The developing therapeutic relationship may lead patients to disclose deeply held concerns and result in emotional release. It is important in this situation to distinguish between sympathy and empathy in response to this cathartic process, maintaining a professional distance, but at the same time feeling comfortable to simply 'be' with patients and their distress (Rahman 2000).

Successful collaboration between patient, professional and family will be influenced by communication issues. In situations where it is difficult to encourage a patient to talk, activity can act as a catalyst, focusing on something other than the conversation and relieving some of the tension (Ainscough 1998). Difficulties with communication may be related to sensory problems such as poor hearing or sight, cognitive impairment, or difficulties with language (dealt with in detail in Ch. 12). An understanding of cultural differences and the significance of particular beliefs and practices will enable the professional to know what questions to ask in order to provide appropriate care (Neuberger 2004).

In some cultures, death is a taboo subject, where stoicism and hiding emotions is more acceptable than discussion. Decisions may be made by the family, not the individual, and people will want to spend time with their family, which might make it difficult to see the patient alone. Health professionals must have respect for the value systems of different cultures, such as modesty (Sikhs and Hindus), and being at peace with God (Muslims), and recognise the importance of family-related activities such as the rituals around food and religious days, for example family meals on the Jewish Sabbath. In Chinese societies, people tend to live in extended family groups and so do not need to be independent. However, in today's society, the grandparents may have a childcare role and so the necessity to be able to perform domestic activities is still appropriate. Using the life-story model to uncover cultural issues (Chochinov et al 2005), involving the family and being aware of the family dynamic, will all help ensure the individual nature of that particular group, within the context of their own culture.

Collaboration in palliative care involves not only the patient, but the wider family group. This can lead to difficulties when the relatives or carers have a different perspective from those of the patient and believe that the patient should have different goals, sometimes insisting that these should be aimed for. Other staff may support this view, but it is important to elicit the true priorities for the patient and to adhere to these. It may also be impossible to facilitate certain goals within the limitations of the workplace. Equipment may be too expensive or inappropriate, or patients may be too ill to comply with the carer's wishes for example, and in this situation the reasoning behind the professional's decision must be made clear, with alternative, achievable suggestions put forward. In this way, the professional will act as the patient's advocate, ensuring that they will not be made to feel useless, more disabled and more of a burden on the family.

Assessment

Initial assessments in the form of specific models of practice will identify need and therefore provide a baseline for interventions, but frailty will affect the patient's ability to comply for any length of time with this process (Periyakoil et al 2005), and although this method will be instructive to the professional, it will serve to highlight how much the patient cannot now do, a situation that may be challenging to the individual. Palliative care assessment needs to acknowledge the individual's losses, but at the same time, highlight the remaining positives. This may involve suggesting changes in how previous occupations are carried out, or focusing on possible new activities (Bye 1998). Many people still want to maintain their independence, even in the face of such debilitating disease, but they can be directed towards developing this control in new areas that will still bring meaning and satisfaction to their lives. A sensitive approach will uncover the reasoning behind their choice of activities and allow suggestions to be made as to how they could use their limited energies for doing something that they consider more pleasurable, e.g. talking to friends, having their hair done, being creative.

People need to be given permission *not* to do the things that they have considered part of their lifestyle for their whole lives, and to have 'me' time, for example not dressing themselves means having energy to speak to friends on the phone, etc. Involving the family in the assessment process will reveal what they are willing to do to help. It is important to consider the need to assess the ability to dress, feed or bathe themselves of those patients who are happy to accept this support from someone else who is willing to do it – either the nurse in the inpatient unit, or a carer at home.

Rapidly changing situations mean that assessments need to be ongoing and flexible, and may not be relevant even the next day. Pre-empting deterioration and introducing coping strategies before issues arise – being one step ahead – will help to avoid feelings of hopelessness and despair at the increasing limitations imposed on that person's lifestyle and perpetuate feelings of control. However, the time required for formal assessments makes their repeated use prohibitive. Patients would need to use their limited energies for the assessment and not to participate in the activities that are important to them, contradicting the advice given to do what is important to them and ignore everything else. Tuning into the patient, the family and their needs by observation, watching and listening for cues, and encouraging sharing of the patient's personal narrative will be a very effective means of continuous assessment in these circumstances (Clouston 2003). Those involved with the well-being of the dying need to be creative and find different ways for people to use their own words to describe their situation, their perspective of themselves and the wider influence of their illness, not only on themselves, but on those closest to them.

The narrative method offers a further insight into the patient's world and can be used as an adjunct to basic assessment techniques, giving a wider picture and a deeper understanding of the situation, leading to an enhanced and holistic view. The story will develop throughout any interactions with the patient – during the assessment process, activity sessions, activities-of-daily-living assessment and practice, creative activities, group sessions, relaxation, and other healthcare duties such as bathing patients, changing beds, applying dressings, drug rounds, etc. (Clouston 2003). Encouraging the telling of personal stories will also offer subtle clues about cognitive ability, relationships, fears, and the influence of emotional issues on symptoms, enhancing the understanding of who that person is and how the illness impacts on the person's lifestyle. It will raise the professional's awareness of cultural and ethnic influences and help with the understanding of the rituals and traditions influencing the roles of individuals within the family (Chochinov et al 2005) and how the illness has affected that unit as a whole.

Another method of assessment that should be considered is communication through the senses. This is particularly useful with children, and is referred to in Appendix 12.4.

Enablement

As the disease progresses, preoccupation with physical abilities is superseded by a growing awareness of existential issues (Foley 2004) and a recognition of the importance of relationships. Goal setting takes on a different perspective as people face the inevitable changes to their previous life plans. Their goals are constantly shifting, as their perception of themselves and their future is dramatically and irreversibly altered and they begin to make their spiritual and mental preparations for death (vanderPloeg 2001). The physical constraints imposed by the illness make them increasingly dependant, and they face an altered future with new priorities needing to be made in the face of limited time and physical and mental resources. Goals may reflect previous occupations and roles, which are not only related to paid employment, but perhaps to previous activities that gave patients pleasure and satisfaction, and will represent their social and emotional status and, consequently, their relationships.

At this transitional stage in a person's life, the ratio between continuity of 'normal' lifestyle and completion of tasks related to the end of life will gradually change. The focus of goals shifts towards the fulfilment of hopes and wishes precious to the individual and may involve revisiting certain times in the past in order to re-evaluate these experiences and perhaps deal with issues that are still outstanding from that time. By addressing any unfinished business in this way, patients can feel that emotional closure has been reached, and that they can let go of this life, feeling that they have achieved their goals. Professionals can offer support to patients, by helping them to redetermine their goals, and supporting and directing them in the achievement of these goals, thereby maintaining a sense of personhood and control. This is a challenging role for the professional, but the establishment of new, different goals, roles and routines will ensure that patients still feel productive, competent and motivated and that their integrity and self-esteem will be maintained (Boog 2006).

How people are perceived by others, and having some influence over that view, can be an important goal in palliative care. Patients are aware of how their appearance and physical and mental abilities have been affected by their illness or its treatments, and want those around them to know what they were like before. Personalising their environment with photos, press cuttings, poems, paintings, etc. or telling their life story are ways of achieving this, as is having some control over their activities of daily living (ADLs) and their appearance.

A further concern when people are dying, related to who they are and who they have been, is how they will be remembered, if at all. When people focus on the future, their goal is to have their memory live on through the generations, and for others to see that they have made a positive mark on life. Relationships increase in importance at this time and projected anger and its repercussions on a relationship may make the goal one of finding and offering an explanation for their behaviour, and achieving reconciliation (Cassidy 1991) in order that they will be remembered the way that they want to be.

When people's expectations of themselves do not match their physical or mental abilities, and the goals that they set themselves are unachievable, introducing sub-goals is a viable option (Bye 1998). These can highlight positive achievements along the way, promoting a sense of success. Poor levels of physical function can be countered with activity on a cognitive, decision-making plane where goals can still be achievable, just approached from a different perspective. In this situation, the therapeutic relationship and the trust that it instils, is an important factor in patients feeling that they are still participating and controlling the situation. Multidisciplinary involvement in working towards such goals will provide ongoing acknowledgement of the patient's efforts, giving a greater chance of success and continued participation in the activity.

In the same way that the illness experience is subjective, so too is the experience of well-being. Measurement of outcome in palliative care can be viewed from the perspective of patients, their carers or staff, and any conflict between a patient's choice of goals and that of others involved will have some influence on the result of any intervention (Needham & Newbury 2004).

For the professional, review meetings, reflection meetings (Prochnau et al 2003) and multidisciplinary meetings will all provide staff with the opportunity for evaluation and perhaps realignment of patient goals, and the feedback from relatives and carers either verbally, during the patient's admission, or in the form of letters and cards after the patient's death, will be an indication of their satisfaction with the service.

In view of the fact that goals in palliative care will be client-established, even if they are not fully achieved because of deterioration and death, the process of goal setting will, in itself, be therapeutic as it will be perceived as a positive experience by patients (Bye 1998, Prochnau et al 2003). Their continued compliance will further confirm the acceptability of the intervention, and ongoing assessment will ensure that the focus of their goals remains appropriate.

The measurement of successful outcome to activities will be directly related to the unique goals of the individual patient. People will choose to pursue these goals in a variety of ways, changing direction, or being guided by the professional as necessary, in direct response to their past and present life trajectory and the issues that influence that. Continued participation and the drive to pursue their goals can be accepted as a measure of successful outcome in these circumstances.

A poor outcome will be indicative of unrealistic goal setting on the part of any or all of the people involved, and a rapid reassessment of the situation will be necessary in order to avoid demoralisation and lack of hope. It may be the result of a low self-esteem and fear of failure, poor symptom management or an inability to recognise personal limitations. Outcomes may also be compromised when the patient is a poor historian, and so matching that person with appropriate activities could be problematical, or there may be a basic lack of understanding of the concept, as in those with learning difficulties. However, for some people, non-compliance is linked to adoption of the sick role, which will have given them power over their situation and a status that they may be unwilling or unable to relinquish. Lack of participation, disinterest and boredom mean that it is time to change direction, employ lateral thinking and move forward. Or it may be time to say 'stop' and allow the person just to be.

Perhaps, then, the best measure of a successful outcome will be found in the expert opinion of the patient, and within that, the best indicating factor of successful outcomes will be the accomplishment of discrete goals and the satisfaction that the patient gains within that achievement.

Problem solving

Problem solving in palliative care is a multifaceted activity, involving clinical reasoning skills, an empathic relationship and the ability to assimilate a diverse range of information into a holistic picture before deciding on the most appropriate course of action. A thorough understanding of the complete situation, from the patient perspective, will also indicate how people can be involved in their treatment (Mattingly 1991). This response is further enhanced by the use, either consciously or unconsciously, of previous experience that may be personal or professional, or both (Norman 2003).

Intuition, or the art of problem solving, is the ability to sift through the information available and to frame the present situation within the wider picture of people's lives, enabling them to move forward with dignity and hope. The complex and subjective nature of the dying experience means that there is a unique set of problems for each individual, and therefore, a unique array of solutions. Patients may not fully appreciate their limitations, and so professionals may find that they are juggling what the patient wants to do with what is possible. Thinking laterally, and using creative solutions are positive ways to deal with this seemingly impossible situation, as is responding to the urgency with which some patients feel driven to complete certain tasks (de Hennezel 1997).

Non-compliance with treatment programmes can be due to several causes. Patients with low self-esteem may fear failure, or the choice of activity may be inappropriate, due to sparse information being made available, including the influence of issues that remain undisclosed. Symptom management may be poor, or patients unable or unwilling to recognise their limitations, physically and mentally.

Using activity as a therapeutic tool

At times of transition, such as the diagnosis of life-threatening disease, being able to participate in previously meaningful occupations can restore a sense of control into people's lives (Rahman 2000, Vrkljan & Miller-Polgar 2001). Adaptation of activities and a flexible treatment plan will ensure that the activities are still manageable despite fluctuating abilities. The use of planning, pacing and prioritising during activity sessions in the hospice, and practising relaxation techniques, will introduce patients to these concepts and encourage them to adopt the idea at home. The provision of leaflets as back-up will help ensure both patients' and carers' understanding of the techniques, offering a means of control by enabling them to actively participate in their own treatment. It is important to remember to negotiate how much people want to know when giving information to patients and carers.

Continuing with a past interest or activity can be unsatisfactory, however, as people may no longer achieve an acceptable result, but by listening to their story and understanding why particular activities have meaning for them, it may be possible to introduce other, different pursuits that will be equally satisfying.

Fatigue and poor concentration are major considerations, leading to the boredom that is often experienced by the terminally ill. Discovering that they can still learn to participate in new and enjoyable activities can help alleviate this, giving structure to the day and resulting in a more positive self-regard and an improvement in perception of quality of life. Positive feedback given during and after the activity will ensure there is continued motivation to continue with the activity.

Activities can help in the control of a variety of unpleasant symptoms, including pain (Rahman 2000), particularly when these are influenced by stress and anxiety, providing distraction by encouraging concentration (Holland 1984). This is not to be confused with diversion and trying to make people feel useful (Tigges & Sherman 1983), but rather offering useful coping strategies that can be implemented at home. Some people already use particular coping strategies, and listening to the narratives of their lives and their illness will help deduce what these are and how and when they are used.

Where patients have very limited resources, making any form of physical activity unachievable, professionals need to help them change the emphasis of their view of themselves from that of a 'doing' person to one of a 'being' (Kissane et al 2001). The stories that people tell in the course of activities may develop into life review, a positive and meaningful exercise that may help them find closure (Rahman 2000).

As the disease progresses, people tend towards activities influenced by relationships and emotional ties. For the patient, these may involve looking at the tasks of grief and bereavement – externalising thoughts and feelings by writing letters, cards and poems, making gifts and memory albums, or enjoying a particular pleasure one last time, e.g. having a meal together with a loved one on the veranda of the inpatient unit. Activities based on leaving legacies are often goals for the last few weeks of life and need to be simple and easy to produce, and quick to finish.

Interventions often have to be unique, each basic activity having a different slant to make it client centred and individual to that person. Control in activities of daily living means more than personal care at a basic level. It can include shopping for new clothes and make-up, indulging in beauty treatments and massage, and helping people to feel good about themselves. Personhood and body image are interconnected, and recent literature recommends that every interaction with the patient should be seen as an opportunity to underline personhood (Chochinov et al 2005) whether it is during the assessment process, or carrying out interventions.

Some people find it difficult to relax, or to think of themselves instead of others, and need to be given permission to be self-indulgent, to be inactive and just 'be'. It is important for the professional to maximise the time when patients are lucid and have the energy to concentrate, by being flexible enough to see them when they are able, and allowing enough time for the preparation and finishing of creative items. Diminishing resources mean that an increasing amount of help will be needed to complete the task, but care must be taken to ensure that these activities are carried out in such a way that patients feel it is their project. When people can no longer engage in activity on a physical level, participation in a passive way can be used successfully to maintain a sense of meaning in their lives.

Activities might be based around people wanting to give something back to those who have cared for them. They may feel they are a burden, or that they want to thank those who have been attentive during their illness.

For some relatives, sitting at the bedside can be a difficult and lonely time. They want to feel useful and will often ask for knitting, or may want to help the patient with craftwork. They can be encouraged to help with information for diaries, life stories and memory albums, or they may want to try some creative activities together with the patient. It can also be suggested that they might like to help the patient choose a book, tape or video, or read out the television listings and help choose the programmes for the day.

Group work

Group activity in palliative care encompasses a wide array of choices, in response to the varied and changing needs of the patients. The aims of the group should be relevant to the needs of all of the participants, including those with sensory and cognitive limitations, and should engender a sense of achievement – often experienced as praise from others (Dawson 1993). A supportive (Holland 1984) and accepting social environment will encourage social interaction between the members of a group (Williams 2002) where developing empathic relationships enhance a sense of belonging, counteracting feelings of social isolation (Dawson 1993). By participating in a shared activity, and responding to the needs of the other members, for example by helping a new person to feel part of an existing group, people feel that they can make a useful contribution (Holland 1984, Lyons et al 2002).

As interpersonal skills improve, people begin to feel more confident about expressing feelings, and sharing experiences with others, reflecting on their present situation and its context within their lives (Lyons et al 2002). Fears and frustrations may be discussed (Dawson 1993) and feedback from others in the group may help towards the discovery of inner strengths and a greater understanding of the self. Boredom and loneliness can be replaced with friendship and feeling confident and comfortable enough to accept that sharing humour, fun and enjoyment is not only still appropriate, but a useful coping mechanism (Adamle 2005).

Group discussion related to the management of activities of daily living, such as planning, pacing and prioritising, and practice of relaxation techniques all help with group cohesiveness, as the participants recognise more common issues to link them together; and freedom to choose whether or not to participate in a group session will enhance feelings of independence and control. Patients who do not actively participate do feel that they are making a contribution to the group dynamic by merely being there (Lyons et al 2002) and, for some, being able to observe the group activity in order to see what happens, will give them the confidence to join in later. At times, people may be seated with the group, but be working as individuals within that context, concentrating on their own projects and only interacting with the rest of the group occasionally. In this way, they can still benefit from the group situation, but can choose to 'opt out' when they want.

Activities may be the catalyst for discussion within the group, whilst conversely, conversation amongst group members may provide the support that some people need to learn new skills and discover new talents (Lloyd & Maas 1997, Lyons at al 2002).

Activities suitable for group work may include reminiscence, baking, glass painting, silk painting, or collage.

Environmental adaptation

Support of the patient and the carer can be enhanced by the provision of appropriate and timely assistive equipment, enabling optimal functioning and creating a sense of control (Rahman 2000). Communication difficulties may be addressed by using a Loop system, both for individuals and for a group with compromised hearing, and can be effective for people with no hearing aids as well as those who use them. Non-verbal systems for those with communication difficulties should also be made available, and these are described in Chapter 12. Where limited physical power and diminished mental ability are issues, alternatives to the switching systems available on the nurse call systems, such as touch pads and buttons, are easily obtainable and can help to reduce anxiety.

Magnifiers, improved lighting, positioning and providing adaptive devices such as cutlery and pen grips will further enhance the sense of regaining some degree of control.

References

Adamle K N 2005 Humor in hospice care: who, where, and how much? American Journal of Hospice and Palliative Care 22(4):287–290

Ainscough K 1998 The therapeutic value of activity in child psychiatry. British Journal of Occupational Therapy 61(5):223–226

Allied Health Professions Palliative Care Project Team 2004 Allied health professional services for cancer-related palliative care. An assessment of need. Online. Available: www.palliativecareglasgow.info/pages/ahpproj.asp

Andrews J 2000 The value of reflective practice: a student case study. British Journal of Occupational Therapy 63 (8):396–398

Boog K 2006 The use of creativity as a psychodynamic activity. In: Cooper J (ed) Occupational therapy in oncology and palliative care, 2nd edn. Wiley, London, pp 175–187

Bruera E, Schmitz B, Pither J et al 2000 The frequency and correlates of dyspnoea in patients with advanced cancer. Journal of Pain and Symptom Management 19(5):357–362

Bye R 1998 When clients are dying: occupational therapists' perspectives. Occupational Therapy Journal of Research 18(1):3–24

Carter H, Macleod R, Brander P et al 2004 Living with a terminal illness: patients' priorities. Journal of Advanced Nursing 45(6):611–620

Cassidy S 1991 Terminal care. In: Watson M (ed) Cancer patient care: psychosocial treatment methods. BPS Books, Cambridge, p 147

Chochinov H, Hack T, Hassard T et al 2005 Dignity therapy: a novel psychotherapeutic intervention for patients near the end of life. Journal of Clinical Oncology 23(24):5520–5525

Clouston T 2003 Narrative methods: talk, listening and representation. British Journal of Occupational Therapy 66(4):136–142

Corner J, Plant H, Ahern R et al 1996 Non-pharmacological intervention for breathlessness in lung cancer. Palliative Medicine 10:299–305

Creek J 2003 Occupational therapy defined as a complex intervention. College of Occupational Therapists, London, pp 29–30

Dawson S 1993 The role of occupational therapy groups in an Australian hospice. American Journal of Hospice and Palliative Care 10(4):13–17

Dawson S, Barker J 1995 Hospice and palliative care: a Delphi survey of occupational therapists' roles and training needs. Australian Occupational Therapy Journal 42:119–127

de Hennezel M 1997 Intimate death: how the dying teach us to live. Warner, London

Foley G 2004 Quality of life for people with motor neurone disease: a consideration for occupational therapists. British Journal of Occupational Therapy 67(12):551–553

Holland A E 1984 Occupational therapy and day care for the terminally ill. Occupational Therapy 47:345–348

Kissane D W, Clarke D M, Street A F 2001 Demoralization syndrome – a relevant psychiatric diagnosis for palliative care. Journal of Palliative Care 17(1):12–21

Lichter I 1991 Some psychological causes of distress in the terminally ill. Palliative Medicine. 5:138–146

Lichter I, Mooney J, Boyd M 1993 Biography as therapy. Palliative Medicine 7:133–137

Lloyd C 1989 Maximising occupational role performance with the terminally ill patient. British Journal of Occupational Therapy 52(6):227–230

Lloyd C, Maas F 1997 Occupational therapy group work in psychiatric settings. British Journal of Occupational Therapy 60(5):226–230

Lugton J 2002 Communicating with dying people and their relatives. Radcliffe Medical Press, Oxford, p 122

Lyons M, Orozovic N, Davis J et al 2002 Doing–being–becoming: occupational experiences of persons with life-threatening illness. American Journal of Occupational Therapy 56(3):285–295

Mackenzie A, Beecraft S 2004 The use of psychodynamic observation as a tool for learning and reflective practice when working with older adults. British Journal of Occupational Therapy 67(12):533–539

Mattingly C 1991 The narrative nature of clinical reasoning. American Journal of Occupational Therapy 45(11):998–1005

National Institute for Clinical Excellence (NICE) 2004 Improving supportive and palliative care for adults with cancer. NHS Guidance on Cancer Services. NICE, London

Needham P R, Newbury J 2004 Goal-setting as a measure of outcome in palliative care. Palliative Medicine 18:444–451

Neuberger J 2004 Dying well: a guide to enabling a good death, 2nd edn. Radcliffe Publishing, Oxford, pp 105–106

NHS Scotland 2004 Allied Health Professions Research and Development Action Plan. Scottish Executive, Edinburgh

Norman G 2003 The role of experience in the development of clinical reasoning. Editorial. International Journal of Therapy and Rehabilitation 10(11):488

Nowak K B, Wandel J C 1998 The sharing of self in geriatric clinical practice: case report and analysis. Geriatric Nursing 19(1):34–37

Periyakoil VS, Skultety K, Sheikh J 2005 Panic, anxiety and chronic dyspnoea. Journal of Palliative Medicine 8(2):453–459

Prochnau C, Liu L, Bowman J 2003 Personal– professional connections in palliative care occupational therapy. American Journal of Occupational Therapy 57(2):196–204

Rahman H 2000 Journey of providing care in hospice: perspectives of occupational therapists. Qualitative Health Research 10(6):806–818

Scottish Intercollegiate Guideline Network (SIGN) 2000 Control of pain in patients with cancer. (Guideline no. 44) SIGN, Edinburgh

Tanaka K, Akechi T, Okuyama T et al 2002 Factors correlated with dyspnoea in advanced lung cancer patients: organic causes and what else? Journal of Pain and Symptom Management 23(6):490–500

Tigges K N, Sherman L K 1983 The treatment of the hospice patient: from occupational history to occupational role. American Journal of Occupational Therapy 37(4):235–238

vanderPloeg W 2001 Health promotion in palliative care: an occupational perspective. Australian Occupational Therapy Journal 48:45–48

Vrkljan B, Miller-Polgar J 2001 Meaning of occupational engagement in life-threatening illness: a qualitative pilot project. Canadian Journal of Occupational Therapy 68(4):237–246

Watson J et al 2006 Barriers to implementing an integrated care pathway for the last days of life in nursing homes. International Journal of Palliative Nursing 12(5):234–240

Williams B 2002 Teaching through artwork in terminal care. European Journal of Palliative Care 9(1):34–36

World Health Organization (WHO) 2004a Better palliative care for older people. WHO, Denmark. Online. Available: www.euro.who.int/

World Health Organization (WHO) 2004b Palliative care – the solid facts. WHO, Denmark. Online. Available: www.euro.who.int/

Impact

Claire Tester

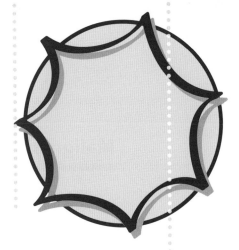

Rock a bye baby on the treetop,
When the wind blows the cradle will rock,
When the bough breaks the baby will fall
And down will come baby, cradle and all.

Nursery rhyme

Key words

emotional and psychological impact; distress; grief; helplessness; malignant
and non-malignant conditions; understanding in childhood and adolescence;
guilt; members of the family

Chapter contents

2

When a child or adult is diagnosed with a life-limiting condition, the prognosis is often given at the same time. The emotional and psychological impact of a life-limiting condition is profoundly distressing; life can no longer be the same. The normality of everyday life is shattered. Longaker (1997) writes that when her husband was diagnosed with acute leukaemia, 'My legs suddenly buckled underneath me . . . feeling as though the world was collapsing around me.' There is shock and grief. There is uncertainty as to what will happen and how life will change, what lies ahead and the fear of the unknown. There is hope that a treatment may be found which will halt the progression of the condition, or even a cure found. Thoughts of death are often accompanied by anxiety and panic: the fear and dread of separation of parent and child, of loved ones, and of life itself. The impulse to survive and to live drives each of us from birth and remains with us until we accept our dying. To have to be faced with one's own mortality is to come to terms with the enforced separation and letting go of loved ones, of this life, and body. There is a not knowing what will happen and when. The unspoken is of death and dying. There is a helplessness experienced by loved ones, as well as the person affected. In this chapter the impact for the patient as child, young adult and adult will be considered. The impact upon the family will also be discussed, as well as the role of palliative care at home and at hospice. An overview will be given regarding malignant and non-malignant conditions in palliative care and how these impact differently.

Malignant and non-malignant conditions

Malignant conditions refer to the different types of cancer. Cancer occurs across the age spectrum and can present acutely. Some cancers are more difficult to detect in the early stages, which can lead to a late presentation as in lung cancer. Cancer occurs in healthy children and adults. There are different types of cancer, i.e. they occur in different parts of the body and may be benign or malignant and may have different rates of growth. Cancer can present as an acute condition that can be successfully treated if diagnosed and treated at an early stage, and if it is accessible and responsive to treatment. The diagnosis of cancer for many is still associated with death and dying and instils fear and anxiety. However, cancer has a high incidence of survivorship. In palliative care, cancer patients are referred because the cancer is not responding to treatment or is too far advanced. Children, young adults and adults with cancer which is treated and then in complete remission may be given the all-clear after 5 years. They may be regarded as having a long-term condition that will need constant self-monitoring and may reoccur – or it may not. Someone with terminal cancer, which is still being treated, may be referred for palliative care. The cancer may be inoperable, unresponsive to active treatment, as advanced primary or secondary cancer. It is important to understand the cancer journey that people have been on, where they are along the journey, and what they understand. For example, the person may have received radiotherapy and chemotherapy which has been unsuccessful, or may not have received these because of presenting at an advanced stage. The situation can change from being acute to palliative.

Occupational therapist: 'One day we were talking to a young woman about her treatment, and the next day after her scan result, we were having to address palliative care options. The difference of 24 hours and the change in our approach was dramatic. She was so distressed.'

To be referred for palliative care is an acknowledgement that the cancer is not curable (Pappas 2005). Non-malignant conditions include conditions that are genetic, inherited and life-limiting, which Goldman & Schuller (2001) identified as:

- metabolic disorders, e.g. mucopolysaccharidoses such as Sanfilippo
- diseases of the nervous system, e.g. Batten's disease, Duchenne muscular dystrophy
- diseases of the respiratory system, e.g. cystic fibrosis
- chromosomal disorders such as Edwards' syndrome
- disorders of the skin and subcutaneous tissues, e.g. epidermolysis bullosa
- disorders of the immune system, e.g. Wiskott–Aldrich syndrome
- diseases of the cardiovascular system such as cardiac myopathy
- organ failure, e.g. liver or kidney.

These may be diagnosed at birth or in early childhood. The child and the parents are taken along the course of the condition and a referral for palliative care may be made at a stage when either significant deterioration has occurred, or support is needed for the family and child or young person. In this way children may be known to a children's hospice and palliative care services for years. Degenerative conditions are often long term chronic disorders that reach a stage of deterioration which requires palliative care. This usually affects adults rather than children. Conditions include heart failure, and respiratory difficulties such as emphysema. The person will have been living with the condition for some time, and be referred for palliative care when the terminal stage of the condition is approached. Care may be received at home through a community palliative care team, or in a hospice. As some adult hospices have day care facilities, patients may attend the hospice for day care, being admitted for the terminal stage only. The choice to die at home with support is not universally available, as it is dependent upon the community services available and the ability of the family to act as full-time carers.

Children as patients

Infants and children are usually not told of their condition but their experiences throughout diagnostic tests, visits to clinic, examinations by different people and blood tests all indicate to them that something is not right. The anxiety and attention of the parents and relatives adds to the suspicion that something is *really* not right. Infants and young children can become understand-ably insecure and 'clingy' to the parent(s) in the midst of all of this. The age of the child and nature of the attachment relationship is significant when diagnosis and prognosis are made, for the child may have developed a secure, or insecure, relationship with the mother which affects the resilience and sense of security of a child in the midst of so much change. However, all children are aware of a parent's anxiety and also of their own symptoms and pain (see Ch. 3). It is still uncertain whether children should be told they will die. Children's understanding of death varies according to age, ability and experience (see Appendix 2.1).

Children who have cancer have had a normal and usually healthy life until this time. The cancer treatments they will have undergone will have affected them physically, emotionally, psychologically and socially. They no longer look the same, their energy fluctuates, they miss out on being with their peers, and find themselves on a cancer ward with other children at different stages of treatment and with different tumours. Their whole life is different and a hospital routine can become their life whilst on the ward. The treatment is continued so that they can get better. The children who do not get better and become terminally ill may continue to be treated actively, or be referred to a children's hospice. As one mother said as she arrived with her son, 'We tried so hard not to be here, to get to this stage. It's too much.' She tried to hide her sobbing but was heard by her son. He had terminal cancer and died a week later at the hospice.

For children, there is a gradual realisation of how ill they are, which Lansdown (1987) identified in cancer as being in five stages:

1. I am very sick.
2. I have an illness that can kill people.
3. I have an illness that can kill children.
4. I may not get better.
5. I am dying.

Children with inherited non-malignant conditions have been living with their condition and have experienced deterioration, which may have involved developmental delay, decline of motor skills, sensory impairment, communication difficulties or a combination of all of these.

> A boy of 10 years with leukodystrophy was still cognitively and intellectually able but was losing his motor skills and had difficulty communicating.

When the familiar becomes unfamiliar, as one's own body loses its strength and ability, the emotional experience is of profound loss and helplessness, as well as anger and frustration. Children may regress to an earlier emotional stage of wanting the mother, of wanting attention, of being frustrated. This is understandable but not always understood and they are often termed 'difficult' children. When children deteriorate, the changes are experienced as losses and can be bewildering and frightening, further exacerbated by the acceptance of family and staff that this is normal. It is normal for the course of the condition, but not for the child. This creates stress for the child, which builds up and has to find a release that presents as pain and hostility (Weininger 1996).

> A 10-year-old girl with a brain tumour constantly surprised staff with her aggressive behaviour and swearing. It was observed that her behaviour was most aggressive when she wanted to do some activity but did not have the muscle power. It seemed she was becoming increasingly frustrated with her own body.

It is necessary to find out what children understand about their condition. They will often provide cues or even outright questions. It is necessary too to discuss regularly with parents what they think their children understand about what is happening to them, and what the parents have told their children and want them to know. Children with deteriorating conditions which are life-limiting, or terminal, experience social loss of peers and relationships, of social activities and in many ways the normality of childhood.

Young adults as patients

This term includes all the teenage years. During this time there are three distinct stages of adolescence: early, middle and late, which highlight emotional development and behaviour. Adolescence is a time the body changes, developing from a child to an adult, biological changes bringing about psychological changes (Horne 1999). It is helpful to consider the stages of change in brief so that the unique difficulties of an adolescent might be better understood.

- *Early adolescence.* This is linked to the onset of puberty, which does not always start at 13. It may begin earlier at 10 years, or later. There can be anxiety as early adolescents seek to compare themselves in regards to the start of puberty and rates of growth, as everyone is different and asking themselves what is happening and whether it is happening to everyone else. This is a time of uncertainty as the body is changing – development of secondary sexual characteristics, growth of pubic hair, a change of voice for boys, and acne. This can lead to some regression in behaviour in the face of so much change. Indeed the lack of personal hygiene at this stage is linked to the embarrassment of change.
- *Mid-adolescence.* Relationships are close in mid-adolescence with same-sex friendships moving to group friendships. Withdrawal from the parents and family is common as the adolescent seeks the 'optimal safe intimate distance . . . to accommodate change' at this mid stage. Trying out different clothing styles and activities contribute to the seeking of an identity. This is also linked with the sense of the future as an adult (Jarvis 1999). There is a potency of sexual energy at this stage, which can be frustrating. There are educational pressures of

examinations and discussions about career possibilities, leaving school or continuing in higher education involving success or failure in results. This is stressful. Added to this mix is falling in love, and the pain of rejection. There is an awkwardness at this stage because, while it embraces the end of childhood when toys are discarded, adulthood is still distant.

- *Late adolescence.* This final stage spans 17 years through to age 20. It is marked by leaving school and the family home for work or higher education and independence. There is an increased pressure to achieve academically if in higher education. There are also financial pressures, whether in work or in higher education, which can result in incurring debt.

From these stages of adolescence it can be seen that identity formation (Jarvis 1999), sexual identity and physical growth are key experiences. Unless this is acknowledged fully, a hospital or hospice environment can deny independence and freedom. Even though the young person might be physically weak and perceived as being incapable of much activity, choice and expressing individuality are forms of freedom that need not be squashed. For the adolescent with a life-limiting condition there is an arrest of the normality of development, which can be accompanied by depression, or anxiety. For some, there is an abandonment of self-regard and self-care: as one 16-year-old braking harshly in his power wheelchair remarked, 'I'm going to die anyway.' The sense of isolation and despair may be hidden, but exists. Parents may understandably be overly protective, which can affect the emotional development of a young person by stifling it or encouraging regression.

> 'I sleep next to him in a separate bed in his room so that I can turn him in the night when he needs,' said one mother of her 14-year-old son.

21

The emotional double bind of adolescents attempting to protect their parents by not showing their own distress in order not to upset them is remarkable in its generosity but creates a distance for the young people as they perceive themselves to be the cause of their parents' unhappiness. This still leaves the adolescents with their own feelings of distress. The emotional development and experiences of the young adult need to be considered fully, as often young people in their late teens are referred to adult services where admission to an adult hospice is often with much older patients, or younger adolescents may be placed with younger children. Young adults have unique needs as they are neither child nor adult, and whilst coping with growing and developing are experiencing extreme emotional disturbance, as well as the physical symptoms of their condition. They have a drive to try out life as much as they can before it is lost.

Adults as patients

Being referred for palliative care forces one to confront one's own mortality. In cancer many contemplate this already at diagnosis and when undergoing treatment, but there is always hope that treatment will work and that the cancer will be eradicated. When required to consider one's own mortality, one asks who is ready for this? Very few of us. This is the challenge in palliative care.

A mother writing after her diagnosis and prognosis of terminal cancer: 'I meet my child from school. I feel a little numb and distant as if looking at my life from the outside. As my son tells me his news I hold on tightly to his hand. I cannot hear him properly because I am thinking of how much I want to see him grow up over time. I don't know what is going on in my own body and how much time it will give me. As I go into my home I catch myself looking at all of the framed photos, of our child and his Dad, that I have taken but there are none of me. Already I am not there. I want to be normal but feel different. I don't know what to do with myself. I want to be busy. I cannot concentrate. Time on my own feels selfish but I want to withdraw. It is when I am on my own that I wonder how my son will live without his mother, if my husband would remarry. I even catch myself wondering who it would be. I feel alone and foolish with these thoughts. How do I determine what my priorities are? I resolve to make a list but they are all immediate things, tidy up, make a cake. I realise I cannot make long-term plans. My make-up takes longer now when I can be bothered. I start wearing my best clothes as if to get some wear out of them. I receive compliments. My clothes are my armour to protect and make me look as if I am good and whole and together when I am falling apart. I feel a wave of loss of being separated from my husband, my child, my life, of a forced leaving and to a place I have not even considered. Already I want my old life back.'

The impact for this young mother immediately results in feelings of anxiety, and agitation. She recognises her difficulty in being able to plan for the near, and distant, future as she contemplates the possible separation from her child if the treatment is unsuccessful. This leads to her fear of the child growing up without her, and both losing a shared future. She is already becoming aware that she will not feature in her family's future. She has not yet considered the loss of her future self, or her own health needs, but is feeling the *present* loss of normality.

The age of people and their stage in life can affect their acceptance of the prognosis.

A man of 87 years remarked: 'Well I have had a good innings and lasted more than the 3 score years and 10. I have a lot to be thankful for in my life as I look back on it.'

It is not always the case that an older person might be more ready to accept dying; the prognosis and referral to palliative care can tip some into a depressive state from which they may not have time to recover. The phrase 'turning one's face to the wall' is appropriate when adults feel there is nothing more that can be done for them, and they wait to die. The idea of being ready to die and to let go of this life and loved ones can be dependent upon many things, such as healing past hurts, sharing family secrets, or seeking religion. This relates to one's own story of one's life, one's own narrative and a visiting of any emotional wounds received or inflicted.

The family dynamics are affected especially if the person requires care at home. The spouse or adult children may support the caring at home, which may be for an extended period. This can cause strain and tensions amongst a family. The situation can be manipulated by family members for their own ends, with tactics of 'just do this or it will upset Mum'.

Parents of affected children

The role of parents is generally understood to protect and nurture a child through infancy, childhood and into adulthood, but parents of a child with a life-limiting condition often feel they are no longer able to keep their child safe and free from harm.

> An 11-year-old boy with Duchenne muscular dystrophy said: 'My dad says he is in a war. A war with my condition. He says he wants to fight it and beat it and stop it. I don't know if he can win.'

Parents can become frustrated by the need to protect their child, as if through their own efforts they might be able to shield the child from illness, as if through their lack of effort they are at fault. As one mother said, 'I feel so guilty. I cannot keep her safe.' This is particularly relevant to cancer when it is felt that something has been missed or not spotted soon enough.

> Mother of 14-year-old son: 'He said, "When I comb my hair I have a spot." "It probably is a spot, son, or a mole," I said. "Don't worry about it." As time went on he came back and said, "You know I think that spot has got bigger." Well I looked at it and it was a lump. He had thick curly hair and it wouldn't really be noticed. He washed his own hair you see.' The boy died from a brain tumour with spinal metastases. The mother could not forgive herself for not having spotted it sooner or understanding it.

Cultural and religious beliefs of parents can affect their reaction to their child's condition. For many parents there is a sense that they are being punished, or hurt by their god. Some parents may also experience a guilt as if they have passed on a 'faulty gene' and may be somehow incomplete as individuals themselves. A mother said, 'When he was diagnosed after birth I looked at him and thought what has happened? Where did he get that from? Is it my body that has done that?' One father with a boy with a life-limiting condition said, 'It is all my fault.' Genetic testing had proved there was a link with the father's side of the family. Aspects of inadequacy, guilt and failure can appear quickly. As one couple remarked, 'We can only make faulty babies.' Parents perceive themselves as passing something 'bad' or harmful on. All of these aspects of guilt and sense of failure create intolerable stresses upon the parents as individuals and on their relationship (Grinyer 2002). The financial implications of taking time off from work, and of costs of travelling to and from hospital as well as the extra expense of special purchases take their toll. Family and friends do rally round but find it hard to sustain the amount of support as time goes on. The accumulated strain upon the parents builds and they can feel very isolated, as well as physically and emotionally exhausted. The accessing of understandable and relevant information from medical staff can increase the sense of helplessness too. Parents try hard to remain calm and cooperative with staff when their feelings may be of frustration, sometimes believing that staff are withholding information. Waiting for appointments or to see the doctor, and sitting in a hospital or hospice can seem endless. 'My life is not my own any more,' said one mother, 'I might as well get a job here.' The combination of these stresses together with trying to cope with the demands of other children, or dependants, as well as the needs of the affected child, result in an overwhelming burden which at times is totally impossible. Parents need support in many different ways, practical as well as emotional. In many ways parents need looking after too, so that they can better care for and support their child. The role of grandparents may fulfil part of this need, but they are often severely impacted upon themselves. For grandparents there is a double impact: of their grandchild's condition, and of their own child's (the parent of the child) pain. This is often accompanied by a guilt that they should have the terminal condition rather than their offspring, as this is the accepted world order (Tester 2006). This can compound the helplessness felt by the grandparents.

Children of affected parents

When an adult is a parent requiring palliative care, the child or children can have real difficulty in understanding what is happening. This depends upon the age of the children and what they have been told, and further what they understand about what they have been told. If it is a non-malignant condition, children will be aware of a parent's condition although may not know it is life-limiting. For terminal cancer there may be a short time in the parent moving from being well to becoming ill through side effects of the treatment, to the terminal stage. Young children can feel omnipotent and that they might have caused the death of a parent through perceived naughty behaviour. As one young woman admitted, 'When my mother died I was 5 years old and I thought it was because I had not eaten my vegetables and not brushed my teeth properly. It took me ages to realise it was not my fault.'

As discussed earlier, parents protect children, but if they appear to succumb to something harmful and fall ill, then they can no longer continue this protection and keep safe the child who is not as strong as the adult.

An occupational therapist recalled a 4-year-old child who always carried a toy gun and a small sword with him: 'He would wave them at the staff to keep us away. His mum said he even slept with his weapons every night. Whilst small boys ordinarily have swords and guns as part of play, this child was using these as weapons for defence and perceived protection 24/7. He appeared as a little "toughy" but was a very vulnerable and frightened child.'

In an attempt to protect them from seeing a very ill parent, children may be kept away and looked after by someone else, because the other parent, if there is one, can be full of grief, and may have difficulties coping. This can further distance children and add to the confusion they may feel. If children or young people live with a single parent who is terminally ill, this can create even further emotional distress, for they may have to live with an estranged other parent or with an appointed guardian. In either situation they lose the familiarity of their own home and of the family life as they knew it. If this necessitates a move to another geographical area, there may be further losses of their school and friends. For some children this disruption and loss occurs before the death of a parent and they can be seen to suffer several losses, or bereavements.

When parents are dying the 'children' may be adults. The impact upon these people of their parent's terminal illness depends upon several factors: their relationship, whether they are dependent upon the parents in any way, their own age and stage in life and past bereavement experiences.

A young adult who has left home for university, a middle-aged woman who has her own home and family, and an older adult in his 70s whose mother is dying are examples of different adults at different stages in their own lives. These 'children' are often actively involved and may adopt the parental role of caring for their ill parent, and providing support for the other parent (Parkes et al 1999). This is difficult and can become complicated.

> Daughter aged 29 years: 'When Mum was so ill it was as if I was the mum, washing her face, helping her to sit up, spoon-feeding her at one point as if she was a child. All the time I wanted to be reassured and looked after as I was so upset, and I was already missing Mum. Dad needed so much looking after, he wasn't eating properly or looking after himself. I had to move back in for a bit. They both suddenly seemed so vulnerable and childlike, both needing looking after but in different ways. My husband was so supportive and helped me so much, I don't know how I would have managed without him. He looked after me.'

Here the daughter recognised the change and dependency of her parents upon her, and her role changed. The loving and supportive relationship she had with her husband provided the security and care a parent might have fulfilled for a child in the attachment relationship. Some adults may be dependent upon their parents in different ways such as living at home with both or one parent for years with no intention of leaving. This includes adults with learning difficulties. Consequently the relationship may be very close and the impact upon the adult can echo that of a child, or a spouse.

Siblings of affected children

When well siblings have a brother or sister with an inherited life-limiting condition they have not known anything different. However, their degree of acceptance of the attention and extra care their ill sibling requires from parents is not universally accepted nor understood. A child who has terminal cancer suddenly becomes ill, and life changes. For the sibling in real terms this may mean that after-school activities cannot be continued, that they may be shuttled to different houses after school, or stay with relatives. Life is not the same. On top of this the child who has had the same upbringing and parents is seriously ill. This raises the fear that the sibling too may become ill or have the same condition lying dormant and hidden. These thoughts can result in anxiety, and be seen in behaviour.

> One sister aged 7 years would never eat any food produced by the hospice kitchen. She saw her sister eat it and although her parents and others ate too she would refuse. Her mother spoke to her about it and it seemed she thought it was food for 'sick' children. She maintained this abstinence for a year until her sister died.

Bluebond-Langner (1996) identified the stigma attached to chronic and terminal illness which is felt by the whole family and the care for the ill child at the expense of the well child. There may be outward signs to the home of disability such as a ramp to the door, or a designated parking space which can be 'distinctly uncool' for the siblings (Tester 2006, p. 113). There is evidence to suggest that well siblings may emotionally regress (Lindsay & MacCarthy 1974), and display hostility (Burton 1975). However, there may be positive and adaptive changes which occur (Kramer 1984) such as the development of altruism, and compassion. It depends upon the communication within the family, the relationships and parenting, the ages of the children and the progression of the condition, and understanding of the well siblings, plus the normality which is maintained for the well siblings (Bluebond-Langner 1996). Siblings as adults can experience the guilt of 'there for the grace of God go I'. This can create a sense of relief, as well as an anxiety that the same condition may occur later for them. This echoes the feelings of younger siblings.

The impact upon staff is discussed in Chapters 13 and 14. See Chapter 3 for impact on relationships; Chapter 11 for the importance of narrative in making sense of impact; and Chapters 7 and 12 for counselling and active listening.

References

Bluebond-Langner M 1996 In the shadow of illness – parents and siblings of the chronically ill child. Princeton University Press, New Jersey

Burton L 1975 The family life of sick children. Routledge, London, p 198

Goldman A, Schuller I 2001 Children and young adults. In: Addington Hall J, Higginson J (eds) Palliative care for non-cancer patients. Oxford University Press, Oxford

Grinyer A 2002 Cancer in young adults. Open University Press, Buckingham

Horne A 1999 Normal emotional development. In: Lanaydo M, Horne A (eds) The handbook of child and adolescent psychotherapy. Routledge, London

Jarvis C 1999 Adolescence and the search for identity. In: Hindle D, Smith M V (eds) Personality development – a psychoanalytic perspective. Routledge, London

Kramer R F 1984 Living with childhood cancer: impact on the healthy siblings. Oncological Nursing Forum 11(1): 44–51

Lansdown R 1987 The development of the concept of death and its relationship to communicating with dying children. In: Karas E (ed) Current issues in clinical psychology. Plenum, London

Lindsay M, MacCarthy D 1974 Caring for the brother or sister of a dying child. In: Burton L (ed) Care of the child facing death. Routledge, London, p 193

Longaker C 1997 Facing death and finding hope. Arrow, London, p 3

Pappas G 2005 Concepts to reality – anthropological perspectives on palliative care. Online. Available: http://www.hab.hrsa.gov/publications/palliative/anthroplogicalperspectives 4 Nov 2005

Parkes C M, Stevenson-Hinde J, Marris P (eds) 1999 Attachment across the life cycle. Routledge, London

Tester C 2006 OT in paediatric oncology and palliative care. In: Cooper J (ed) Occupational therapy in oncology and palliative care. Wiley, London

Weininger O 1996 Being and not being – clinical applications of the death instinct. Karnac, London

Suggested further reading

Beyond Indigo 2006 Developmental stages in a child's understanding of death or loss. Online. Available: http://www.beyondindigo.com 4 Nov 2006

Brasch M, Keen B 2006 Common reactions to grief/loss. Online. Available: http://www.notmykid.org 2 Sept 2006

Kastenbaum R 2006 Children and adolescents' understanding of death. Online. Available: http://www.deathreference.com 4 Dec 2006

Kemp C, Allen S 2006 Children – how children view dying and death. Online. Available: http://www3.baylor.edu/~Charles_Kemp/terminal_illness/children.htm 2 Sept 2006

Lawson M J 2005 On understanding and helping children process death. Online. Available: http://www.grief.com 1 November 2006

People Living with Cancer (PLWC) 2005 Helping a child or teenager who is grieving. Online. Available: http://www.plwc.org 2 Sept 2006

SIDS Mid-Atlantic 2006 Children's understanding of death. Online. Available: http://www.sidsma.org 4 November 2006

Appendix 2.1
Children's understanding of death and dying

Claire Tester

Adults, that is parents and relatives, understandably avoid talking about death and dying to a child when a sibling or parent is terminally ill (Bretherton 1999) in order to protect the child, and perhaps because they find it difficult to accept themselves.

> As one child aged 8 said: 'It was when Mummy was crying and shouting at Daddy that Robert was dying that I heard about it. I was upstairs in bed, but I could hear her. They didn't know I heard.'

Children are often described as 'resilient', and 'able to bounce back and carry on' as if the child who is left has somehow got over it, or is not emotionally affected in some way. This is not true, it is just that the child employs ways of coping with the emotional trauma of the loss but cannot process it fully. It becomes part of the emotional make-up of the child and like a cork can surface at a later stage. Children's needs are not less than those of adults but adults can have difficulty coping with them, especially a parent who is grieving for the death of a child or spouse. Adults in a caring role for other adults do not see the child as having needs in the same way.

Here are some thoughts on providing some support to children whose siblings, or parent has died, which are from my own experience.

Children can have real difficulty in understanding and accepting the finality of death: someone who was breathing, alive and living, has been turned off in some way. This is understandable when every week cartoon characters and TV superheroes spring back to life. Questions asked include: Where has the person gone? What happened? Are they in a deep sleep? Adults' explanations of the person having 'gone to heaven', 'with the angels', 'gone to be a star in the sky', or even 'gone away to live with Jesus' are taken literally by young children and are misleading. Children may be helped in their bereavement, depending upon their level of understanding and how they were prepared for what is, and will be, happening. It is understandable that such discussions are painful for parents, who also anticipate the distress and upset that this knowledge will cause the child, but children fill in gaps in their knowledge with their own fears which can be very frightening. It is as if the monster-under-the-bed becomes real and can become overwhelming. This includes the fear that *they* will die at some point in their childhood, or the omnipotent belief that a sibling's or parent's illness is attributable to them directly. The age and corresponding developmental stage of the child are significant to the child's understanding and acceptance of someone dying.

Here is a brief overview of abilities to understand and comprehend:

Infant to toddler (3 years)

If there is an attachment relationship with the adult then it is not death but separation which is understood, and it is indeed like a death, a disappearance and loss of the adult. This can be experienced as distress, and searching, followed by a clinging and reattachment to another close carer. (This relationship should ideally have been developed before the death of the parent.)

If a sibling has died there is a sense of missing the person if there was a close and playful relationship.

Even though infants or toddlers are so young, they will be sensitive to feelings and moods of others around them without understanding why. Routines can be lost or change. This can lead to clingy behaviour, or attention-seeking actions.

3–6 years

Like hide-and-seek, the person is hidden from view but will appear, so that death is not permanent, only temporary. This thinking is reinforced to a degree when adults speak of 'seeing the person again in heaven' or feeling that the person is still present, just not as visible. Such concepts are not understood. Children think in concrete terms and look for the person to appear. The child can believe the person to be asleep like Snow White or Sleeping Beauty, and it is a matter of finding the right way to wake the sleeper, which they see as logical, just no one has thought of it.

> John (age 5) stood on the bed as his dead brother lay in it. 'Wake up!' he shouted. He pulled at his brother's hair. He turned the tape music up very loudly. Exasperated he went over to his brother and pulled his eyelashes to wake him.

Children are aware that something is very wrong and can become fearful, e.g. bed wetting, clingy behaviour, worried about going to sleep themselves, and too of other family members going to sleep. Sleep can be linked with dying, through past experience or the way an adult uses euphemisms. For example a pet dying may go to the vet to be 'put to sleep'. Children at this age have difficulty not just explaining how they feel but understanding how they feel. It feels like everything, so all the parts are muddled up and that is how they are. This leads to an involuntary acting out in behaviour and play. Children may even appear aggressive. The world as they know it has fallen apart, and adults around them appear to be crumbling and crying. Children need lots of reassurance although things cannot be the same, nor mended.

6–9 years

At this age, there is an understanding that death does occur, but at a distance. If it is close it can be personally threatening. There is questioning of what, how and why did it happen, which can seem relentless in children's attempts to understand. This can also include questioning of themselves, which may be kept quiet: Did I make it happen because I was cross with her? I got fed up with the wheelchair and not going to the park, wishing he wasn't there, did I wish him away? Was there something I could have done? These are very troubling questions, which are linked to guilt that can stay lodged with the child. It can be difficult for the child to voice these thoughts too, as by speaking them to another the fear is that they may be confirmed by the adult.

Adults often make what they believe to be encouraging comments to children of this age: 'Lucky Mum's got you to look after her', and 'You'll need to be a big boy, you're the man of the family now'.

It is the child who is vulnerable, needs looking after and feels like regressing to an earlier age and stage of being looked after and kept safe.

9–13 years

This age marks the start of intellectual thinking, being aware of the scale and size of the world, and one's place in it. The child has a clearer understanding of death and dying, of a body's systems shutting down and ceasing to function. Emotionally the child is developing a sense of independence and of wanting to appear grown up. For some children, puberty has begun and they may look older. This appearance of looking older and more solid is misleading, as they are still vulnerable and beginning to form a sense of their own identity. There can be embarrassment and a wishing to hide the bereavement from peers. This can affect relationships. One child explained that he did not want other children upsetting him about the death of his father at school. He was worried that he would cry and get upset. This could only lead to taunts and being treated differently.

This leads to an attempt to keep grief private. It can be reinforced by a sense of not wanting to cause or trigger further distress to the parent. In addition this understanding of death raises fears and anxieties that the child might have inherited the condition, or be infected, or may be due a fateful accident. Such fears can remain kept and hidden for years. Children can believe that the parent has not imparted such facts to them as it would be distressing for the parent. Such fears can also be projected about the parent(s), and that the child will become an orphan.

Grieving needs to be accepted as normal in the home. The child needs to be able to cry and have questions answered, and some anticipated in a sensitive and loving manner. This can be difficult for parents who are angry at the death of their child or spouse.

> The mother shouted at her son: 'Of course you haven't got it! *You're* OK.'

13–18 years

As young people, adolescents are often perceived as being adults, with an adult's acceptance of death and grief reaction. They may feel they have to act as adults and 'keep everything in', not being witness to an adult's distress. A father admitted he did not want his 17-year-old daughter to think 'he'd lost it', so did not get upset. By not speaking of his wife in front of his daughter he felt able to gain control of his distress to an extent. His daughter admitted that she could not cry in front of her father as 'he never cries, and might think it pathetic'. She found it hard that he did not mention her mother. When discussing this with a therapist, they both admitted trying to 'be brave for the other'. There is an honesty required. Depending upon age, and the relationship the adolescent had with the deceased, the reaction and acceptance can vary. The adolescent may have been going through a difficult time, invoking negative thoughts such as, 'He never liked me anyway.' This can lead to regret, or guilt, and confusion.

Throughout all ages and stages it is important to understand and recognise that children and young people are affected by the death of a loved one. The key things to remember are:

- To be honest. Not to use euphemisms which a child takes literally.
- To consider the level of understanding of the child. This means that as the child grows older more questions will be asked to help with understanding. This is important but can seem puzzling to an adult.
- Children are sensitive to what is going on around them, including the moods and behaviour of adult(s). This affects the child.

- The younger the children the more important routines and normal patterns are when the world has changed in their eyes. This alone is not enough, the main caregiver needs to nurture the child.
- Encourage and accept discussion of the deceased. This person has been an important person in life and needs to be assimilated into the present as part of the narrative in a positive way. Photograph albums can be helpful here, especially an album for the children or young people, with pictures of themselves and family too.
- Opportunities for expression. Not everyone can identify their feelings especially children. Painting, drawing, clay modelling, making things, can be used as positive outlets for expression. It can be helpful to talk about it: 'Tell me about your picture', rather than put your own views on it, 'That looks like a boat, or is it meant to be a house?'
- Honesty becomes more important as a child grows into a young person, for without openness and honest reliable answers, questions are no longer asked.
- A tolerance of negative behaviour is necessary but it needs to be recognised for what it is, that the child or adolescent is having difficulty understanding, coping and coming to terms with the death.

Anticipatory bereavement by the affected child is discussed in Chapter 6.

Reference

Bretherton I 1999 Updating the 'internal working model' construct: some reflections. Attachment and Human Development 1(3):342–357

Attachment and relationships

Claire Tester

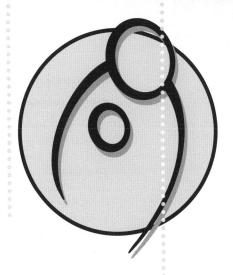

'I live with the Lost Boys.'
'Who are they?'
'Why, they are the children who fall out of their perambulators when their nurses are looking the other way. If they are not claimed within 7 days, they are sent far away to the Never-Never-Never Land.'

J M Barrie *The Story of Peter Pan*

Key words

separation; family dynamics; emotional experience; internal world; behaviour; secure and insecure; containment; anxiety; loss; infant; child; adult

3

There is anxiety and fear associated with the diagnosis and prognosis of limited-life conditions. The reflective piece in Chapter 2 (p. 22) illustrates something of the distress when confronting one's own mortality. To consider dying in this world is to leave one's life and loved ones behind – a separation. Separating is a parting (Holmes 1993), which implies a connection, a relationship. There are different forms of connections, and of relationships. Our first relationship with mother, or main caregiver, acts as a formative relationship or attachment for relationships with others. An attachment relationship is defined as one concerned with needing and providing protection (Parkes et al 1999). As Parkes et al write, 'out of the infant's first relationship with its mother stems a set of expectations and assumptions which will not easily be changed.' In this chapter attachment theory will be outlined and how it can impact upon relationships and family dynamics. Separation and the emotional experience through prolonged hospital stays will be considered across the age spectrum from babies to old age.

Overview of attachment theory

Attachment and the subsequent experience of separation and loss in the infant/young child can echo down the years to adulthood said Bowlby (1997), for the first relationship we form with the mother acts as a blueprint for all the relationships that follow. Research has given further significance to this first relationship and proved it to have far-reaching effects on the emotional internal world of the infant, and on personality development. The areas of neurobiology and developmental psychology have strengthened the importance of attachment and its contribution to psychoanalysis. In 1950 when Bowlby was advising the World Health Organization on the mental health of homeless children he concluded that a warm, intimate and continuous relationship between the young child and its mother, or a main caregiver, was essential for mental health. At this time Bowlby's colleague James Robertson was observing young children experiencing temporary loss of the mother during hospital stays (as parents were not allowed extended visiting time with their children). John Bowlby looked at the theoretical implications of loss and saw that the work linked Freud's (1913) basic tenet that the unconscious can be seen in behaviour through which the emotional life can be understood. Bowlby described the first relationship with the mother as involving 'love and hate, anxiety and defence, attachment and loss' (1997, p. xi). Bowlby wrote of an instinctive behaviour pattern which could be triggered by a stimulus or stimuli which could be either internal, e.g. hunger, tiredness etc., or external, e.g. solitude, loud noises (Hopkins 1999). The aim and motivation of the infant's behaviour is to seek proximity to the main caregiver and with it the perceived sense of security, and to survive. He termed this 'attachment behaviour', and within it saw three distinct phases in response to loss of the mother. These were: (1) separation anxiety (threat of loss); (2) grief and mourning (acceptance of loss); and (3) defence (protection from the pain of loss). Each stage has observable behaviours of: (1) protests and inconsolable crying; (2) intermittent crying and seeking mother; and (3) an acceptance of mother's absence leading to a detached manner. There may be smiles but it is as if the emotion has been exhausted. Even when the mother returns after this last stage has been reached, there has been the loss of something of real value in the emotional tie between the child and the mother. Bowlby (1997, p. xiii) described the young child missing his mother as being like a 'hunger for his mother's love and presence as great as his hunger for food'. This attachment is vital to the child for physical survival, and reveals an emotional dependency upon the mother which could be perceived as a form of emotional sustenance and nourishment. Bowlby said that adults could still be disturbed by traumatic experiences of separation and loss in early life.

> A woman of 65 years commented: 'I cannot bear to be without my husband or one of my daughters with me at any time. I cannot bear to be on my own. My husband wonders if it's due to my mum dying when I was 3.'

Bowlby (1997) identified different behavioural responses to breakdowns in attachment relationships as leading to emotional disturbances and the forming of certain personalities such as dependent and hysterical, affectionless and psychopathic. Research into different areas of attachment behaviour has led to the development of attachment theory for understanding behaviour and identifying emotional responses. Mary Ainsworth (1969) observed different patterns of behaviour between mothers and their infants which determined the nature of the attachment, looking at the quality of the attachment or 'tie' to the mother and the degree of sensitivity between mother and infant which affected the attachment relationship. She identified two types of attachment: secure and insecure. Children assessed as having a secure attachment have developed a basic trust (Erikson 1950). Children assessed as having an insecure attachment are 'anxiously' attached, developing one of two defence strategies: avoidant, or ambivalent/ resistant. The avoidant baby shuns contact from the mother, not seeking comfort from her. The ambivalent or resistant infant becomes very distressed by separation and cannot be consoled by mother on her return, presenting as both angry and clingy, being ambivalent towards her. Ainsworth (1970) found that patterns of attachment behaviour were established by the age of 1 year and were closely related to the nature of the mothering the baby received during that time. She highlighted the sensitivity of the infant to the mother and vice versa. This work was extended to older children by the Grossmanns (1986) at 6 years and again at 10 years using the separation anxiety test to show that attachment patterns of infancy remain. Mary Main (1999) introduced the 'adult attachment interview' in which parents are asked to talk about their childhood relationship with a parent. Main and her fellow researchers found that there were patterns indicating either a secure or an insecure attachment relationship with a person's own parent which was often being actively repeated with that person's own child. This traces back to Bowlby's own assertion that the first relationship can be repeated through life with other close relationships. When there is a good enough relationship all is well but the consequences of negative experiences can impair the neurochemical responses, which in turn affect the emotional and social functioning of an individual (Stern 1998). Negative experiences might include emotional neglect, perhaps attributed to maternal depression, or abuse, both affecting the attachment relationship, which can affect relationships in later life. This was verified by Brown & Harris's 1978 Walthamstow study (1991) linking childhood loss of mother with depression in adulthood. However Klaus Grossmann (1999) holds that nothing is permanent or necessarily fixed, and that language and relationships through life can alter or shape an initial attachment pattern and that 'old' internal working models (IWM) can be replaced with 'new' ones, even in older people (Grossmann 1999). This possibility of change links with aspects of reconciliation, healing and connecting relationships at the end of life, regardless of age.

Thinking about infants and young children

The earliest attachment relationship is important to each of us, and the nature of the emotional tie to the mother is dependent upon the mother's emotional availability and nurturing capacity at the very earliest stage. Psychotherapist Dilys Dawes' view (1999) is that babies do have problems and need help in the early days with their mothers, which introduces the aspect of preventive therapy in attachment, being alert to a difficulty, or potential relationship difficulty, and helping to repair it. How does a life-limiting condition, either for the child, the mother, or the father, affect the attachment relationship? Responses vary but the relationship is affected.

Mother of 3-month-old girl with life-limiting condition: 'I knew what to do with my other daughter but this one is different. She never wanted my milk, and she cries when I pick her up. It's easier not to. She doesn't want me.'

'I feel so guilty bringing this little baby into the world to die. I feel that in her short life I need to put in as much love as I can.'

'I did the night shift and my partner is doing the day shift. We need a break now so are asking for respite for the baby.' Parent of a 10-week-old baby.

'The baby is through there in her cot. She seems happy enough on her own and I just go through when she cries for a nappy change or it's time for a tube feed.' Mother.

'He likes the TV. He just sits there all day, and I get on with things in the house.' Mother of a 5-month-old baby.

The mother could not look at the baby and would turn her head away from the direction of her child. 'She doesn't want it,' said her husband.

In considering mothers and their babies with life-limiting conditions, there is trauma and distress as the mother finds herself in a dichotomy of loving her child and building a secure attachment, and knowing that the child will die and is dying, and of the foreseen separation. This pain of loving can create an ambivalence in the mother. The mother's ability to act as a container (Bion 1984), her ability to respond to the baby's signals and to 'hold onto a baby's distress' (Weininger 1993) can be compromised. Safier (2000) writes that the mother may be so 'stirred up by the infant's demands' that she cannot meet and modify them, to reassure the child, but instead 'adds a quantum of her own fears . . . [which she] sends back to the baby'. The infant is then left with unmanageable feelings and anxieties it cannot reconcile. Some of the mother's unbearable emotions which are felt by the infant may be mourning for the 'normal' baby she had anticipated if the baby is born with a physical or developmental difficulty or has a life-limiting condition diagnosed at birth (see Ch. 6).

Other factors affecting the ability to contain anxiety can include the frequency and length of stay in hospital for the infant, which affect the relationship with the parent(s).

An 18-month-old girl with complex needs had spent almost her entire life in hospital apart from a few days home, a day at a time, accompanied by a nurse. The staff attended to the child's needs and the mother described the child as 'living at the hospital and having the staff as her family'. The relationship between the mother and child presented as insecure–ambivalent. The child was observed as 'detached' with little interest in people around her including her mother, and the nurses.

One aspect not often acknowledged is the acceptance by the parent of the appearance of the child. Children who have genetic life-limiting conditions may have physical differences such as exaggerated features, which a parent is not always prepared for. This can affect mothers in different ways, of wanting to protect the child, or of difficulty in accepting the infant. Kitzinger (1991) describes meeting one's newborn baby: 'when a woman first meets her baby, she says goodbye to the fantasy baby inside her and greets the real one in her arms. This can be a difficult transition for a woman who . . . was sure that the baby would be perfectly formed and a handicap is revealed.' This 'transition time' can be a time of conflicting emotions for the mother, and support and coming to terms gradually are needed. This is known as the bonding time. However, this time can be dramatically affected when a baby is taken from the mother for tests or taken to the special care baby unit.

'I couldn't walk due to the caesarean but I knew I had to get up to the next floor to go and see my baby. I wanted to know what was wrong. I never saw him. I was almost hysterical with fear of what was the matter, what was missing. I just wanted to be with my baby. The staff were telling me to wait. They probably thought I was mad. They didn't understand.'

'The baby was wrapped so well that I could not see how his skull was affected and his limbs were so weak. But holding him like that just then at minutes old, I just wanted to look at him and hold him. To love him. All the other discoveries came later.'

The way in which the mother is prepared for her new baby, and the time she has with the infant can affect the relationship (Ayers 2003). It can be helpful to gently remind the mother that the baby is already familiar with the mother's voice and vibration of sound from being in the womb (Verny & Kelly 1987). This intimacy and connection is helpful (Trevarthen 2001) and can be often overlooked. Stays in hospital or hospices can interrupt the relationship building between the mother and her infant. Babies are attractive and staff can gravitate to them, wanting to hold them. However, when a parent is present it is important to be mindful that it is the mother's baby and that time for mother and baby is precious, and this time may need nurturing itself. This means that staff should metaphorically step back rather than forward. The environment for the mother and baby is important and every effort should be made to create a soft, comfortable and nurturing environment. This can include a comfortable chair, soft light, baby blankets and items, and gentle music. The nurturing environment is for the mother as well as for the baby. For some parents, a member of staff may act as a 'mother' figure for the new mother in recognising her needs for support. Fathers should be included too, and sensitivity in providing support at a discreet but near distance will be needed by both. Fathers tend to act protectively for the mother and baby. Some fathers can perceive themselves as failed in this regard when a baby is terminally ill and the mother is distressed. Some men can absent themselves from the trauma and give themselves a functional role only, such as fetching and carrying rather than engaging with the baby directly. This is a form of coping behaviour.

Separation

The relationships we form through life are based upon the initial attachment relationship with mother, or main caregiver. Thinking of a child or adult with a life-limiting condition, the increased vulnerability and need for emotional support during times of separation from loved ones when in hospital or a hospice are acutely felt. The effects of separation for a mother and baby have been described as 'a mutilating loss of part of the body' (Tustin 1992). The aloneness and fear can be unbearable. The lack of an emotional containment, which was available to the infant and child through the mother particularly, is experienced as a nothingness, a void (Bion 1984). Children, and young adults, who may not have been told of their prognosis, are sensitive to the behaviour and attitude of those around them. This not-knowing and worrying can increase feelings of emotional isolation. Bion described infants as being aware of a nameless dread leading to an emotional fragmenting. Adults in palliative care have described a sense of emotionally 'falling apart'. This is the same free falling of emotions into a void. How can the child or adult gain a sense of being held together, of being contained and understood? Winnicott (1964) describes the 'good-enough' mother as being able to put the baby back together by physically holding the child, and bearing the emotional turmoil to make it bearable. Thinking of children and adults in palliative care, the aspect of the unbearable thinking of death and dying, of separation and anticipated loss cannot be tolerated. How could it be borne? It is not, and reveals itself in behaviour as it is got rid of (Klein 1998). This is entirely understandable, and normal (see Ch. 13). When a young adult or an adult is feeling emotionally vulnerable and needy it can be viewed by others as immature or childish behaviour. To be cared for by others and nurtured is a fundamental need, linking back to the earliest instinct to survive (Balbernie 2001).

> Husband of woman aged 50 years: 'When I went to see her at visiting time at the hospital I was 10 minutes late. She burst into tears and said she thought I had forgotten her.'

Children

The relationship between a child and parent is an emotional one but other factors can affect its being sustained at times of stress. Separation, such as during a hospital stay or hospice admission, can create intense distress and a yearning sense of loss of the parent by the child (Bowlby 1997). Without the presence of the mother, the distress becomes despair, a grief for the loss of the mother. When there is no special person or attachment relationship the child can form, and the time without the mother figure is prolonged, another stage of grief behaviour begins. This is when the child becomes egocentric and all relationships and interactions are short lived and empty of emotion and real feeling (Bowlby 1997). Bowlby's work led to provision for parents to stay with children at hospital.

> As one mother said, of her 3-year-old: 'My husband and I took it in turns to sleep and wash so that there was always one of us with Ben (child). Ben was frightened by some of the hospital procedures, and the staff kept changing so things always seemed different as everyone seemed to have a different way of doing the same things. We just wanted to be with him to reassure and not let him worry. It helped us too. We all felt better just being together.'

Children seek their parents' protection, but this can be compromised when invasive medical procedures are undertaken or injections and unpleasant medications are administered. When such things happen a young child can perceive that the parents are colluding with the staff. This can be painful for a parent, who can be emotionally torn.

Nurse: 'The father would always sit with his 4-year-old daughter when the time came for his daughter's medication through the porta cava. She would cry and he would hold her on his lap. He always had tears in his eyes too. The mum used to have to go out as she couldn't bear it.'

Children whose parent is terminally ill can experience prolonged breaks in their relationship. Although they are not the affected patient, they are affected, and their sense of being emotionally contained and supported can be overlooked as attention is given to their physical needs, i.e. someone to meet them from school, prepare a meal, and have clothes ready. School teachers may be aware of the situation but seldom have the emotional resources to recognise or meet a child's needs, perceiving this to be a private matter. Addressing the emotional needs of the children or grandchildren of a dying relative are not addressed as a matter of course by adult hospices.

Adults

As adults, the relationship formed with a partner or spouse can be perceived as an attachment relationship. This may be secure or insecure. It is hoped that it is a mutually supportive and emotionally caring relationship, but not all relationships are this way. The nature of the relationship is stressed by one being terminally ill. This is compounded when there is separation.

Wife aged 72 years with terminal cancer and married for 49 years: 'We had spoken about it all for weeks, knowing I was getting worse. I said to John [husband], "You know we can't go on like this. I can't get down the stairs now. I can't do things for myself." I knew it would come to this. We both did. But I said, "I shall need to go into the hospice soon John." He just nodded. We were both in tears . . . just the thought of being apart . . . of not being together . . . and of knowing that there wasn't much time left.'

The attachment relationship between adult partners builds over time, leading to sense of emotional security and stability (Weiss 1991).

Husband 36 years: 'Visiting my wife at the hospice there wasn't any privacy. I just wanted to lie on the bed next to her and hold her. I could only sit and hold her hand. That didn't feel enough.'

Conclusion

Recognising the existence and importance of the attachment relationship, and that there are different kinds, is a way of beginning to understand why people behave as they do when faced by separation, both real on a day-to-day basis and the envisaged separation in death. Putting this in the context of palliative care and of the anticipated separation death brings to each person in a relationship – the fear, loneliness and vulnerability – is to consider how infants, children, young adults, parents and adults can be cared for. It also acknowledges that there is a fear of separation from another, and that anxiety and panic can rise in recognition of this. It is recognised that to be able to observe the attachment relationships of others is to become conscious of one's own, which can be distressing (see Ch. 14). The affect of the fear and nameless dread (Bion 1984) of a life-limiting condition affects the whole family and their perception of being emotionally held and supported. This leaves individuals feeling emotionally exposed and vulnerable.

Below are some suggestions to support relationships:

- Ensure that children, especially young children, are not separated from their mother/main caregiver as much as possible.
- Respect the privacy for hugs and kisses between relatives and loved ones.
- Enable time and family support, e.g. enough chairs, letting people sit on the bed, lowering the bed for children to sit on to see and touch their parent.
- Knock on the door before entering, or stand at the end of the bed to ask permission to carry out a procedure rather than walking straight up to the bedside when visitors are present. Give people a few moments to gather themselves when loved ones leave before administering medication etc.
- Support the person to be at home with loved one(s), even for an afternoon visit.
- Provide easy access to a telephone.
- Encourage people to have familiar items of importance with them (even if such items have to be named).
- Support and enable parents to be with ill children overnight.
- Children take comfort from family photographs in a small album, or plastic-covered photographs of parents for the child to hold. Adults also like to have pictures of family to look upon.
- Discuss photos with children, young adults or adults; this may be comforting when the person in the photograph is absent.
- Find out what reassures a person, regardless of age, especially at night. It might be a small light left on, a favourite story for young children, the phone to call and say goodnight to the person's own children, etc.
- Talk to people when they are without visitors. Check first that they are content for you to talk to them.
- Avoid reprimanding or threatening a child, e.g. 'You had better behave today/be a good boy/girl today, I don't want to tell your mummy you have been naughty/be brave and don't cry today,' etc. These are all to do with the ease of management for staff rather than any compassionate regard for the child or young person's own emotional experience.
- Consider the immediate environment in respect of pillows, duvet cover, blankets, bedside light, and the view available to the person in the bed. Also some thought should be given to the view the visitors have of the person, and the room itself, e.g. it is reasonably tidy, the person is covered up and 'decent', drink is accessible, etc. The general environment should be conducive to the well-being of the people or children using it. This includes colours, light, noise levels, furnishings and views outside. The use of colour can be helpful in creating moods and emotions (Gimbel 1994).
- Touch is important to all human beings, and the lack of it is isolating and reinforces a sense of being separate and set apart from others. Because of political correctness and an overzealous approach, the sensitivity of appropriate touch for another, such as on the hand, or holding the hand, can be denied to someone in want or need.

- Suggestions in the chapters on creativity (Ch. 8), communication (Ch. 12), and narrative (Ch. 11) contribute other ways of supporting and helping to connect the members of a family as they face the inevitable separation of dying.

References

Ainsworth M D, Bell S 1970 Attachment, exploration and separation: illustrated by the behaviour of one year olds in a strange situation. Journal of Child Development 41:49–67

Ainsworth M D, Wittig B A 1969 Attachment and exploratory behaviour of one year olds in a strange situation. In: Foss B M (ed) Determinants of infant behaviour. Methuen, London, vol 4

Ayers M 2003 Mother–infant attachment and psychoanalysis – the eyes of shame. Brunner-Routledge, London

Balbernie R 2001 Circuits and circumstances: the neurobiological consequences of early relationship experiences and how they shape later behaviour. Journal of Child Psychotherapy 27(3):237

Barrie J M 1965 The Story of Peter Pan. Bell & Sons, London

Bion W 1984 Second thoughts. Karnac, London

Bowlby J 1997 Attachment and loss, 2nd edn. Pimlico, London, vol 1

Brown G W, Harris T O 1991 Loss of parent in childhood, attachment style, and depression in adulthood. In: Parkes C M, Stevenson-Hinde J, Marris P (eds) Attachment across the lifecycle. Routledge, London, p 235.

Dawes D 1999 Brief psychotherapy with infants and their parents. In: Lanyado M, Horne A (eds) The handbook of child and adolescent psychotherapy. Routledge, London, p 261

Erikson E 1950 Childhood and society. Norton, New York

Freud S 1913 Further recommendations in the technique of psychoanalysis (on beginning the treatment). In: Rieff P (ed) 1978 Freud; therapy and technique. Macmillan, New York

Gimbel T 1994 Healing with colour. Gaia, London

Grossmann K 1999 Old and new internal working models of attachment: the organization of feelings and language. Attachment and Human Development 1(3):253–269

Grossmann K, Grossmann K E 1986 Capturing the wider view of attachment: a re-analysis of Ainsworth's Strange Situation. In: Izard C E, Read P B (eds) Measuring emotions in infants and children. Cambridge University Press, Cambridge, pp 124–171

Holmes J 1993 John Bowlby and attachment theory. Routledge, London

Hopkins J 1999 Some contributions on attachment theory. In: Lanyado M, Horne A (eds) The handbook of child and adolescent psychotherapy. Routledge, London, p 44

Kitzinger S 1991 Homebirth. Dorling Kindersley, London, pp 185–186

Klein M 1998 The psycho-analysis of children. London, Karnac

Main M 1999 Metacognitive knowledge, metacognitive monitoring, and singular (coherent) vs. multiple (incoherent) model of attachment: findings and directions for future research. In: Parkes C M, Stevenson-Hinde J, Marris P (eds) Attachment across the life cycle. Routledge, London, ch 8, pp 127–159

Parkes C M, Stevenson-Hinde J, Marris P 1999 Attachment across the life cycle. London: Routledge, p 1

Safier R 2000 When the bough breaks: working with parents and infants. In: Symington J (ed) Imprisoned pain and its transformation. Karnac, London, p 134

Stern D 1998 The interpersonal world of the infant. Karnac, London, p 8

Trevarthen C 2001 Intrinsic motives for companionship in understanding: their origin, development, and significance for infant mental health. Infant Mental Health Journal 22(1–2):99

Tustin F 1992 The protective shell in children and adults. Karnac, London, p 218

Verny T, Kelly J 1987 The secret life of the unborn child. Sphere, London

Weininger O 1993 View from the cradle. Karnac, London

Weiss R S 1991 The attachment bond in childhood and adulthood. In: Parkes C M, Stevenson-Hinde J, Marris P (eds) Attachment across the life cycle. Routledge, London, pp 66–75

Winnicott D W 1964 The child, the family and the outside world. Pelican, London

Appendix 3.1
Thinking about babies

Claire Tester

'A person's a person, no matter how small.'

(Dr. Seuss)

Thinking about the emotional well-being of the infant and how we can develop ways of reassuring and calming a baby raises questions about how babies feel, and how they grow and develop. Babies grow and develop skills and learn about the world around them. We know about their milestones. When they are born they can usually already hear, see, make sounds, make movements and feed. So how has that baby grown? Have there been any influences upon the baby before birth? What happens before the baby is born? The baby developing in utero from 4 months onwards until birth can react to stimuli. By the 4th month, the unborn baby can frown, squint and grimace, and has also acquired basic reflexes (Verny & Kelly 1987). What does the baby hear? The mother's heartbeat, the sound of digestion, the sound of blood rushing through arteries and veins, the mother breathing, and the mother's voice (Chamberlain 2006). Dr Henry Truby Professor of Pediatrics, Linguistics and Anthropology at the University of Miami in the 1980s discovered that babies hear clearly from 6 months in utero, and that they move their body in rhythm to their mothers' speech patterns (Verny & Kelly 1987, p. 7). Truby's work looked at the speech patterns we learn and copy from our mothers but which start before we are born. A child hears other sounds and voices too. In an early study where fathers spoke to their baby in utero using short soothing words, the 'newborn was able to pick out his father's voice in a room within the first two hours of being born' and, if crying, would stop at the sound of the father's voice (Peterson 1979).

Dr Thomas Verny says that even at 4 and 5 months babies in utero respond to music because when they hear it, they calm and relax at the sound of Brahms, and kick and are generally very active at Beethoven. The conductor Boris Brott was asked how he had become interested in music. He explained, 'This might sound strange, but music has been a part of me since before birth. As a young man I was mystified by the unusual ability I had, which was to play certain pieces sight unseen. I'd be conducting a score for the first time and, suddenly, the cello line would jump out at me; I'd know the flow of the piece even before I turned the page of the score. One day I mentioned this to my mother, who is a professional cellist. I thought she'd be intrigued because it was always the cello line that was so distinct in my mind. She was; but when she learned what the pieces were, the mystery quickly solved itself. All the scores I knew sight unseen were ones she had played whilst pregnant with me' (Verny & Kelly 1987).

Thinking back to the heartbeat which is ever present for the growing baby in the womb, a steady boom–boom–boom sound, it is familiar, steady and constant. It provides a sense of calm for the baby. A pioneering experiment in 1960 by Salk on newborn babies has led to the development of the field of birth psychology. He used a tape of the human heartbeat, which was played to a nursery ward of newborn babies to observe any differences in behaviour between babies exposed to the sound, and babies who were not. The results were surprising. The 'heartbeat babies' ate more, weighed more, slept more, breathed better, cried less and were generally more healthy than the control set of babies without the sound of the heartbeat. He concluded that the babies found the heartbeat positively beneficial, that they were emotionally reassured and contented by the heartbeat as if the mother was with them, as if they were still in close proximity to her and not separate. The babies felt secure. The newborn babies were already aware of what made them feel secure and reassured, which would indicate that these responses had developed in the womb.

Thinking about feeling

The growing baby in utero is aware of the mother's strong emotions, whether calming or frightening, because of the biological changes which occur. When a mother is suddenly frightened or worried and her body goes into the fight or flight mode, adrenaline is released in her body and affects the baby so that the baby jumps around too. Similarly, when a mother is calm her baby is gently moving in the womb and appears calm. Before thinking about the relationship a baby forms with its mother after birth, some thoughts about the birth itself and the baby's experience of it follow. The baby has grown in the womb, a space full of warm amniotic fluid, and attached to the umbilical cord, able to swim from side to side and up and down until as the baby grows the space becomes cramped. But still the baby can turn itself by pushing against the sides. There is a reddish-orange glow in the womb, a place with the constant sounds of the mother's voice and heartbeat. Many years ago most babies were born at home and now most babies are born in hospital. There are machines to monitor the heartbeat of the baby in utero. There are drugs for the mother to slow down or speed up the labour, and drugs including an epidural, to lessen or numb the pain. The drugs the mother takes cross the placenta and can make their way into the baby's system too. These are normal births. Some babies born at full term or preterm are taken away immediately to the special care baby unit where they encounter a different kind of space to be in and different sounds, and lights. Their mother and father have to visit them on this unit. The song by the band Athlete described the parents' view of their child in a special care baby unit; 'You got wires coming out, you got wires going in . . . I see hope in a plastic box.' The baby is separated in this way from the mother, and nothing is familiar.

It is helpful to keep in mind that babies are able to remember and are aware before they are born (Spelt 1948). They have a memory for their mother's voice and the enclosed warm space they have been inhabiting is familiar; they can move themselves about and are not helpless in the womb. Also, any difficulties or strong emotions the mother may have experienced during pregnancy may also affect them too, both at the time and as memories of strong negative sensations.

Bonding

The nature of the relationship between the mother (or main caregiver) and her infant is the foundation for the baby's emotional development. In Europe, America or Asia the most common shared activity a mother does when pregnant is to stroke and pat her stomach (Verny & Kelly 1987). The mother is aware of the baby and may talk to it, as well as stroke and pat her stomach as the baby grows, all showing that the mother is thinking about the baby. This is a form of bonding which is intrauterine. We acknowledge that the baby and the mother have been together in the same body for 9 months, hearing and feeling but not seeing each other apart from the ultrasound scan images during check-ups. It is as if there has been a separation and now there is a reunion as the baby is born and both see each other. Newborn babies have 20/500 vision; that is, they can see objects clearly if they are close up but not far away. This shapes their world. It is immediate. They can make out facial features if 6–12 inches away. They cannot take in the whole world and so only take in what they can see – things and people close up. Bonding, the initial relationship of holding and looking intently at each other and being together, occurs within the first 12 hours and from this develops the attachment relationship (see main text of chapter).

Thinking about a baby's needs

A newborn baby has instinctive behaviour driven by both internal and external factors.

As Stern (1998, p. 8) writes: 'Infants begin to experience a sense of an emergent self from birth . . . aware of self-organizing processes'. Internal factors are hunger, tiredness, pain, and feeling cold; external factors are 'darkness, loud noises, sudden movements, looming shapes, and solitude' (Hopkins 1999). When babies are upset they look for one of the attachment figures they have learnt to discriminate, that is their mother or father usually, a familiar figure.

Thinking about babies at a children's hospice

Many of the babies at a children's hospice have a developmental delay and a poor prognosis, and I wonder when the mothers were told – in pregnancy, at birth, or a little while after? This timing can really adversely affect the bonding relationship between the baby and mother. Thinking about attachment relationships too, what happened to the baby and mother in the first few hours and days? It is helpful to find out and to understand how the parent and baby have been separated and what has been experienced by the baby. This allows the parent to share the experience of this time and to identify how they have connected. Helping a mother and baby connect at this time can be painful for the parent who can be both resisting rationally and at the same time feeling a loving duty and pull to the infant.

> One mother explained it was the pain of loving the child so much but with guilt and an overwhelming powerlessness to protect the child from harm. She noticed that the father 'kept his distance avoiding talking, holding and touching' the baby girl for the same reasons she felt.

Thinking of the emotional experience from the baby's view provides opportunity to provide comfort and familiarity as much as possible, for example a heartbeat sound. A parent's voice could be recorded – perhaps a familiar lullaby – which could be used for night-time waking. It is necessary to know what soothes the child, and if songs are sung, which they are. Babies who are very quiet and do not make a sound may have learnt that their needs are not met by their mother/attachment figures. These babies might seem to be disconnected. It raises the question of whether babies feel lonely. This is a disturbing idea. How can they be helped to connect to the main carer?

Thinking about the emotional well-being of the baby in the absence of the parent(s), some activities are:

- Sounds – heartbeat sounds and rhythm; the human voice, not a radio voice singing but a real person talking and singing to them, responding to speech patterns. It is helpful to think about the mother's speech pattern, fast, slow, etc., which can be mimicked to an extent.
- Making most of the baby's movement by assisting with resistance to kicking and pushing movements. This can be done at nappy changing time by not grabbing the baby at the ankles but using one of your hands as a flat palm to push gently against both feet whilst changing the nappy. This affords a little resistance and avoids the baby feeling bound at the ankles.
- Warmth is our first sense (see Appendix 9.1). What does the baby lie on? A 'nest' could be made with a rolled blanket in a crescent shape around the baby's legs to kick and push against. This can also provide a sense of security.
- The importance of milk – one of the baby's earliest reflexes is the rooting reflex to turn and find the nipple for milk. As the baby reaches out to explore in later weeks it is the impetus to

find something to suck, either as food or as reassurance, which stimulates the baby to explore, to take to the mouth, to find what can and cannot be eaten. In this way babies begin to explore the immediate world around them. I've noticed that babies who are tube fed are slower to explore and do not seek to take things to their mouth. They need help to explore.

In conclusion

There are so many more simple ideas that can make a difference to a baby, but they require thought about babies, consideration of the emotional experiences of babies, and thinking and finding out about their own stories, or narratives, so far.

References

Chamberlain D B (2006) The fetal senses – sensitivity to touch. Life before birth. Online. Available from: http://www.birthpsychology.com [Accessed 1st December 2006]

Peterson G 1979 The role of some birth related variables in father attachment. American Journal of Orthopsychiatry 49(2):330–338

Salk L 1960 The effects of the normal heartbeat sound on the behaviour of the new-born infant: implications for mental health. Online. Available: http://www.blackwell-synergy.com 1 Dec 2006

Spelt D K 1948 The conditioning of the human foetus in utero. Journal of Experimental Psychology 3:338–346

Stern D 1998 The interpersonal world of the infant. Karnac, London, p 8

Verny T, Kelly J 1987 The secret life of the unborn child. Sphere, London

Palliative rehabilitation

Claire Tester

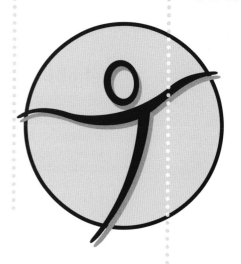

We hold these truths to be sacred and undeniable: that all men are created equal and independent, that from that equal creation they derive rights inherent and inalienable, among which are the preservation of life, and liberty, and the pursuit of happiness.

Thomas Jefferson (1743–1826) Original draft for the Declaration of Independence

Key words

rehabilitation – adults, children and young people; independence; compassion; assessment; pain

4

Introduction

The concept of palliative care originated from the hospice movement but has been a recognised field of practice since 1987 (Hynson & Sawyer 2001) and includes health professionals from different disciplines. It is a new and developing field encompassing all life-limiting conditions, and any age. It is more developed for adult cancer services. However, there are differences and difficulties in interpreting when and where palliative care might begin, and how rehabilitation therapists might work in this area. The idea of paediatric palliative rehabilitation can be harder to define. The World Health Organization (1998) identified palliative care for a child as including the care of 'the child's body, mind and spirit' as well as support to the family. The goal of palliative care is achievement of the best quality of life for patients and their families. Palliative care involves working with children or adults holistically, addressing all of their needs that are unique and personal. The term 'palliative care' carries a meaning of looking after people, caring for them, and 'doing for' them. All of these imply passivity, but palliative rehabilitation encourages a person to be as active as possible, and to be as independent as possible.

Rehabilitation in palliative care

Rehabilitation is understood to restore and to return the ability of a person to function physically, and socially, in their environment, including home, school/higher education, work and leisure activities. This is known well to health professionals who work in rehabilitation. In rehabilitation the traditional model is to work on improving and strengthening skills, leading to independence and discharge from the rehabilitation services. This is relevant to both physical and mental health conditions. However, when rehabilitation is linked to palliative care it is perceived as being confusing and irrelevant as it is associated with improvement and ability. How could it be appropriate or helpful to people with a deteriorating condition which is incurable?

In rehabilitation the emphasis is on achieving one's potential.

Bray & Cooper (2005) identified four types of rehabilitation:

* preventive – to lessen the severity of an existing condition
* restorative – to enable clients to return to premorbid status without significant disability
* supportive – to support the client through decline to remain as functional as possible
* palliative – to assist in symptom control and prevent complications in the advanced stages of a progressive disease.

Rehabilitation does not set out to cure or to always return people to full function in all skills areas, but to support and enable them to live as independently as possible with the condition. In this way it can also be understood as helping a person to readjust to living with a condition, whether it is an amputation, a stroke, a bipolar condition, or a life-limiting condition. Some life-limiting conditions may be regarded as long-term conditions with variable lengths of time. The emphasis of rehabilitation is to enable a person to live as independently as possible, which can involve aids and equipment, coping strategies and problem-solving techniques, and ongoing support. Developing new skills and maintaining existing skills are part of any rehabilitation. In considering the needs of someone receiving palliative care, rehabilitation is helping the person to be as active and independent as possible. This may be reduced to exercising choice when the person may be physically weak, or unable to initiate any movement, or even communicate verbally. Dying is an important stage in life and as one nears the end of one's life there can be much one wishes to do. This is an important time to provide support to enable people to complete the tasks that are meaningful to them, which can include the physical, emotional, social, and spiritual. For example, people experiencing breathlessness on exertion would benefit from a programme in managing breathlessness and fatigue, and guidance on how they can self-manage their energies in order to do what is significant for them. This aspect of 'significance' for the person is fundamental in palliative care rehabilitation, as it is individual to each person. In palliative care rehabilitation there is no set formulaic programme of rehabilitation, as people are different and have unique views on their quality of life.

A man in his 70s with a terminal illness with respiratory difficulty and a general motor weakness wanted to use his energy for his 2-year-old granddaughter's visits so that she might sit on his lap and show her grandfather a favourite book, even though this meant he was so tired that he needed assistance to cut up his food and to eat after the visits. He was aware that he had a small reserve of energy but it was meaningful to him to use it for his granddaughter's visit even though this left him very tired and unable to help himself afterwards.

There can be conflicts in rehabilitation between traditional rehabilitation and palliative rehabilitation because what matters to the person may be at odds with the view and training of the health professional.

Assessing for seating for a young person, Helen, aged 15 years: Helen had a mucopolysaccharide condition and had limited movement, a profound developmental delay, and although unable to speak she could communicate her pain and discomfort, as well as pleasure. The community occupational therapist (OT) carried out a joint assessment with the hospice OT. The community OT was intent on a correct sitting position with 90 degrees at hips and knees, with equal weight distribution at hips and buttocks. This position could not be maintained, as Helen had pain at her left hip (osteochondritis) and as a result would alter her position into extension at her left hip and knee, twisting her body as she did so. Helen's pain relief was effective but she consistently avoided pressure on this area, which her mother thought might be habitual rather than due to pain. The OT considered ways in which the correct position might be maintained, although they would restrict Helen's movement.

The hospice OT was looking for the optimum comfortable sitting position and was guided by Helen rather than a prescribed sitting position. This resulted in a chair which was padded, and could be altered easily into different positions, including tipping backwards and extending the back and seat with lower leg supports and footplate to relieve pressure on sitting. The community OT remarked, 'This isn't the chair or position I would ordinarily prescribe.'

The hospice OT said, 'No but this isn't an ordinary situation.'

The assessment was extensive and considered all aspects, including scoliosis and pressure relief, Helen's preferences for sitting, and her comfort.

Palliative rehabilitation is carried out in consideration of the individual, acknowledging that the person's abilities can deteriorate and change. The rate and degree of change are variable. For example, a young boy assessed for a first wheelchair quickly lost his ability to sit unsupported, including head control, over 12 weeks. He was unable to sit in his new chair. Children in palliative care may be deteriorating and losing skills, but they are growing too. The rate of growth, particularly at adolescence, can be very rapid, so equipment needs to be reviewed regularly. In some conditions a person's energy levels and abilities may fluctuate and vary, with 'good days' and 'bad days'. The emotional state of a person can also have an effect. As one woman, aged 28 years, said, 'Sometimes I have a day when I just feel so low and sad that I just want to cry all day and do nothing. In fact I don't feel like doing anything or seeing anyone. I just can't.'

Planning rehabilitation in palliative care can be a challenge for the health professional (Bye 1998). For OTs and physiotherapists in particular, planning rehabilitation with someone who has a deteriorating condition can be very deskilling for the therapist, because traditional measuring of improvement as a gauge of effective and successful therapy cannot be made (see Ch. 14). The therapists need to change their approach and thinking. The diagram on page 48 illustrates the usual rehabilitation model of improvement and discharge compared to palliative rehabilitation when a person deteriorates, and dies. There are two different directions with a shared starting point, but separate end points. There is a distinct gap, which illustrates the difference in the two approaches and how this gap widens; palliative rehabilitation becoming further and further removed from the familiarity of the normal rehabilitation of improvement leading to discharge. It is in this gap that the therapist can become disorientated and lose direction, leading to deskilling. Therapists who are working on an oncology ward may be faced with palliative care patients at

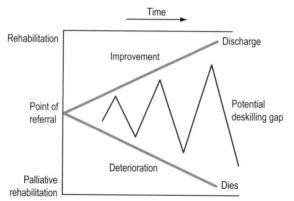

Author's model for potential deskilling of rehabilitation therapists in palliative care.

the same time as patients for rehabilitation and discharge, which both require a different approach. This can be very stressful and demanding.

Rehabilitation in palliative care needs to be reframed by the therapist, as patients may not have any demonstrable improvement in skills (Cooper 2005) and the therapist cannot measure therapy outcomes in terms of progression in strength and ability. Outcomes of therapy need to be measured in terms of enablement, support and quality of life as they relate to the individual and the individual's family.

Assessment and planning, which always involve discussion with the patient, can be a very emotional encounter. As Boog (2005) writes, 'the individual's needs, desires, hopes and fears, goals and ambitions, and feelings of loss may be revealed and the holistic overview will enable development of a strategy to enhance their lifestyle and make it as rewarding as possible'. The therapist needs to allow time for such discussions and to be compassionate. Working with people who have life-limiting conditions is both humbling and emotionally demanding. Listening and guiding people in sharing what is meaningful to them requires time and consideration.

Planning rehabilitation

Usually a condition and the medical intervention received act as a guide to the expected recovery of a person and the therapy intervention required. In palliative care there is no such formula or prescriptive therapy. Everyone is unique, and even when a prognosis is given it can be proved wrong by the patient. As one mother remarked, 'So many times have we been on the verge of my daughter dying but somehow she keeps going and bouncing back.' The starting point for palliative rehabilitation is with individuals, to ascertain with each of them, their level of skill function and difficulties, and what they regard as important and significant for them. Working with children requires an assessment of developmental abilities too. Children and young people have different needs and approaches from those of adults, so are addressed under the heading 'Children and young people', following on from 'Adult rehabilitation'.

Adult rehabilitation

This begins with the person and involves an ongoing assessment of abilities and ascertaining what is important to that person. Depending upon the nature of the person's patient journey there may have been many interviews for essential information and physical assessment. People do become very tired of being asked the same questions, and can feel too that there is no joining up of services and staff when the same information is requested of them. This can be upsetting for them and can affect their level of trust and confidence in a service. Sometimes a summary of interventions is made for the medical file, which can be helpful for the patient and other health professionals. Where possible try to share assessments, e.g. a functional skills assessment, or a discussion of support at home and home circumstances. This may be in conjunction with another health professional, or using a key worker system within the team.

Depending upon the condition, and the service provision, palliative care may be at the terminal stage or may extend for a longer time. For example, children with life-limiting incurable conditions may use a children's hospice for a few years before reaching their terminal phase. The emphasis is upon symptom management and quality of life. Cheville (2000) reports the main concern of palliative care patients as the 'threat of progressive debility and caretaker dependency'. Progressive debility includes increased and uncontrolled pain, and loss of functional and independence skills of daily living leading to an isolation and dependence upon others. The concern of being dependent upon others is linked to the perceived quality of life, which is different for everyone. This usually includes the ability to choose, and to be autonomous (Axelsson & Sjoden 1998). People referred for palliative care may already be feeling helpless and vulnerable in facing their own mortality, but to consider an increased future dependence upon others can lead to a wish to hasten death.

> 62-year-old woman with terminal cancer: 'I'd rather die sooner than have my husband try and do everything for me – feeding and toileting me. It doesn't bear thinking about.'

The therapist needs to be sensitive and develop trust with the patient. The relationship with the patient is central to effective therapeutic intervention. As McCluskey (2005) writes, 'caregivers who can respond with compassion and intelligence and who can support the intelligence and good sense of those who seek their care in whatever state of distress they are in . . . will experience the joy of meeting and being met by a fellow human being'. This sensitivity and compassion are central to the palliative care approach although the core areas of occupational therapy apply (Cooper & Littlechild 2004). These are:

- assessment – initial interview, goal setting, home assessment, cognitive and perceptual assessment, including emotional and spiritual influences on the experience of pain
- equipment – provision, wheelchairs, pressure care
- symptom control – relaxation, fatigue management, psychological support, anxiety management, breathlessness management, splinting, body image, sexuality
- self-care – assessment and practice, transfer assessment and practice
- leisure – leisure activities, creative and recreational activities.

All goals and therapy stem from the therapeutic relationship with the patient and family. Palliative rehabilitation involves patients actively in setting goals and discussing what is meaningful and desired by them. This requires sensitivity on the part of the health professional for a patient may have unrealistic goals. Hope has to be considered here, and a careful and thoughtful exploration in discussion with the person is necessary, rather than dismissing any seemingly unrealistic goals out of hand.

> Mr Brown at 81 was referred for palliative care. He had complex needs, with his main difficulty being emphysema. He was living at home with his wife, aged 75 years, as main carer and support from community nurses. When asked what was most important to him, he answered that he wanted to travel to Canada to see his son. Through discussion, it emerged that he had little contact with his son to whom he wanted to make amends and to heal past difficulties in

their relationship. This was discussed with Mrs Brown, who shared that she had maintained a discreet contact with her son unknown to her husband. With the therapist, both Mr and Mrs Brown were encouraged to discuss and share this information together, and to consider ways for Mr Brown to contact his son directly. This occurred initially through a letter from Mr Brown, and then telephone calls which became regular. The idea of travelling to Canada was quickly dropped by Mr Brown as he was helped to find other ways of connecting with his son.

Independence

Independence can be understood in varying degrees. Traditionally it is understood as being independent in all activities of daily living (ADL), and being able to meet all of one's own needs. However, one's needs can change, and independence may need to be reframed with, and for, each person. For example, independence is relevant to people who may be paralysed and without speech. Their choices and wishes need to be understood and carried out for them. In this way independence can be understood as empowering a person in a dignified and respectful manner. People may be dependent for their physical and ADL needs but their ability to exercise independent will and thinking needs to be considered and encouraged. This is linked to the person's sense of self, spirit, feelings and unique character.

Anger and frustration can occur for someone who loses abilities and skills, particularly in communicating. Different ways of communication can be explored and the person helped. The advice and guidance of a speech and language therapist should be sought, as well as local technology centres for communication difficulties. When a person wishes to express strong emotions and feelings, these should not be ignored but heard and addressed where appropriate. As one father remarked, 'It is difficult to say how upset you are these days to anyone, and let off some steam without being seen to be abusive and difficult.' Emotions run high when there is anxiety and an overwhelming powerlessness when faced with one's mortality. Dying can be a frightening time, and can be lonely for the patient (Doyle 2005). People may be able to adjust and come to terms with their prognosis, which echoes the bereavement process. This bereavement is of their own life and projected possible future (see Ch. 6).

Choice

At times the health professional may see the potential for the person to maintain or achieve certain skills which the patient chooses not to develop. In this situation the agenda of the health professional can be different from that of the patient and conflicting. For people to have choice and options does enable them to opt out of certain therapeutic interventions, which may include medical treatments too. As one nurse commented, 'It was so difficult to witness Tom's obvious pain and deterioration and not be able to do anything about it. He didn't want chemotherapy of any kind, and died in such pain.' This relates back to the importance of the relationship between patient and health professional in being able to discuss and share knowledge and beliefs of the person (Horne 2005). To enable patients to make choice, they need to be fully informed and to understand the consequences of any choices made.

Fatigue is a symptom of cancer and is also seen in other conditions, e.g. heart failure. It involves a lack of energy and a feeling of exhaustion which may be due to chemotherapy, pain, or difficulty in breathing (dyspnoea). Fatigue directly affects the quality of life and restricts choice for a person, impacting emotionally and psychologically, leading to depressive affect (Stone 2002). Fatigue is not always recognised (Krishnasamy 1997).

Fatigue may be prolonged or chronic and can be distressing and disruptive. Therapeutic interventions include fatigue management where the person is helped to plan activity using energy conservation techniques, and relaxation (Lowrie 2006) and psychological interventions such as visualisation and imagery. This can have a positive emotional effect (Siegel 1999) even if the level of physical fatigue level remains unchanged.

Depression and anxiety are perceived as part of the process of dying, and unwittingly reinforced by the family's sense of the hopelessness of the situation (APM 2006). Clinical depression is often undiagnosed and is not treated (Block 2006) because of an overlap of physical symptoms, and an uncertainty of the success of treatment (APM 2006). As occupational therapists are trained in both physical and psychiatric conditions, they should be alert to depressive symptoms, remembering that children and young people can also have psychiatric problems (Cherny 2004, Chochinov et al 1997, Hotopf et al 2002).

Children and young people

Assessment and rehabilitation

Children with life-limiting conditions often have complex needs. Until the mid-1990s work with children tended to be service-led rather than needs-led (ACT 2003). The idea of palliative care for children can be difficult to accept, as it is usually associated with dying. However, palliative care for a child can begin at diagnosis when a prognosis is often made that may be some years hence, or may be intermittent according to the child's need. There is no set pattern for when palliative care begins for a child with a life-limiting condition. It depends upon the need of the child, and the family (see Ch. 2). Thinking about rehabilitation for a child receiving palliative care can also be challenging for health professionals, and it is often overlooked or disregarded.

Therapeutic intervention is requested for positioning, maintaining mobility, and equipment requests in the main. This is also reflected in the care plans which should relate to current assessments of a child's needs including personal care, psychological and emotional support, spiritual support, and education as well as symptom management (ACT 2003).

Paediatric occupational therapist: 'A child aged 13 months had a large file which travelled between home, hospital and hospice. It was called "My care plan for home and hospice". It was a thick file packed with information on medication, when to wash and what to use, administering medication with feeds – and timings for this. There was a section on positioning the child correctly, with pictures. I looked for information about the child's personality, her likes and dislikes, the way she communicated, her developmental level, something about her emotional responses, how she could be comforted, and some of her favourite play. I looked in vain.

'This little girl was registered blind, she ate nothing by mouth so had no oral stimulation, and did not take anything to her mouth to explore, as she could not initiate any movement.

'Although her care plan was completed, shared amongst staff and medically accurate, it was for the staff. The child appeared not to do anything, so she didn't. There was so much to offer this child by way of communicating through touch, developmental play, stimulation and responding to her in a meaningful way, which had not been considered.'

There is a limited view that palliative care for a child is physical care, managing physical symptoms especially when the child is sick and ill. Play is used as a diversion or an occupation. It is assumed that the parents will know what to do for their child and provide whatever is necessary. This is true, to an extent. Children change according to their condition, they can deteriorate and lose skills.

Mother: 'I don't know what to do. I go into the toyshops and want to get something for her, but I can't see anything. She has changed so much. I usually buy something and she cannot use it. I need help.'

Nurse: 'The mother just keeps him on the bed, or puts him in the buggy. She will play with her older child a bit, but I think the mother doesn't know what to do. He doesn't respond to her playing or her voice.'

A child receiving palliative care is still a growing child. Such children's developmental stages will often be affected, even delayed, and there can be deterioration and lost skills. Some of these skills can be maintained, and other skills learnt. Regardless of whether the child is able to communicate or not, initiate movement or not, and has impaired senses, the child or young adult is an emotional being with thoughts and feelings. For some children their physical growth might be arrested but there is still development. Care plans should relate to current assessments of a child's needs including personal care, psychological and emotional support, spiritual support, and education as well as symptom management (ACT 2003). A care plan should reflect good palliative care in meeting all of a person's needs, no matter how young the person is (see Appendix 4.2).

Pain

Dame Cicely Saunders, who led the hospice movement, introduced the concept of 'total pain', which includes physical, psychological, emotional and spiritual pain (Saunders 1993). Although physical pain is recognised and treated, it can be harder to identify emotional and spiritual pain. Understanding the multidimensional properties of the pain experience and its subjective nature is complex. Listening to someone's story and teasing out the important aspects that are influencing the person's well-being requires patience and skill. Pain which remains unresponsive to all efforts to address it by medication, positioning, supplementary equipment, or suggested adjustments to lifestyle management, should be explored in order to uncover a deeper meaning. People may be unaware of the significance of certain contributing factors to their pain, such as relationship issues, loss and lack of control of their situation, and so are unable to find respite from their pain. There are some for whom the illness experience gives them status that perhaps they did not have before. For these individuals, maintenance of the sick role is very important, and they may resist all attempts to find a solution to their pain.

Children and pain

It is understood that all children and infants can experience physical pain, but less understood is that children can also have emotional and psychological pain. Symington (2000) writes that when emotional pain is not recognised it becomes 'imprisoned and hidden' and becomes 'lodged within the personality'. Identifying pain still proves difficult, with pain going undiagnosed and untreated (Twycross 1998). Winnicott (1964) described children as having emotionally intense experiences which can distress and alarm them, dominating the child's whole being. How can a child who presents in such pain be understood? The Royal College of Paediatrics (1997) recommended, 'if the child is not in pain but anxious, a sedative drug may be sufficient'. This acknowledges that pain might not be physical but that the emotions can be managed through sedation. This is one way of managing distress, but it does not address the child's emotional needs nor contribute to the child's emotional well-being. In fact it can create fear in children, who may then anticipate being sedated rather than heard when they voice their upset. As infants and children may not be able to articulate their fears, it does not mean they do not have anxieties and worries. Young adults include mid- to late teenagers who are 'caught' between childhood and adulthood and can have real difficulty in expressing their emotions. For many, communicating pain in its different forms can be impossible if they are unable to communicate actively, and/or are developmentally delayed.

When thinking about the importance of providing 'psychological medicine' (Weininger 1996), it is necessary to consider the emotional experience of the child. When a child *feels* upset this can lead to physical symptoms of distress, e.g. difficulty of breathing as they sob, stomach ache felt through anxiety, and headache too if there are unwanted thoughts. Fatigue, and confusion as a result of treatment or condition, can disorientate and upset a child, so familiarity and reassurance are important. Weininger (1996) suggests an emotionally containing setting where children feel they are understood. This echoes the need to be 'held' emotionally in the thinking of another so that they may no longer feel vulnerable and unsafe (Bion 1967). Without this emotional containment, difficult emotions and feelings are carried by the child alone, and may also be added to by the anxieties projected unwittingly by the mother into her child (see Ch. 3). In practising the ethical principles of respect for individual autonomy, beneficence, non-maleficence, and justice (Randall & Downie 1999), the infant or child's own style of comforting needs to be identified to contribute towards a positive emotional experience for the child. (A 'Home from Home comfort map' is described in Appendix 4.3.)

As Kubler-Ross (1983) wrote, 'during the first few years of life, each child needs a great deal of pampering and nurturing. And so it is with terminal illness'.

References

Academy of Psychosomatic Medicine (APM) 2006 Position statement: psychiatric aspects of excellent end-of-life care. Online. Available: http://www.apm.org/papers/eol-care.shtml 2 Dec 2006

ACT Association for Children with Life-threatening or Terminal Conditions and their Families 2003 A Guide to effective care planning – assessment of children with life limiting conditions and their families. ACT, Bristol. Online. Available: http://www.act.org.uk 25 Oct 2006

Axelsson B, Sjoden P O 1998 Quality of life of cancer patients and their spouses in palliative home care. Palliative Medicine 12(1):29–39

Bion W 1967 Second thoughts. Selected papers on psycho-analysis. Heinemann, London (reprinted 1990, Karnac, London)

Block S 2006 Psychological issues in end-of-life care. Journal of Palliative Medicine 9(3):751–772. Online. Available: http://www.liebertonline.com 2 Dec 2006

Boog K 2005 The use of creativity as a psychodynamic activity. In: Cooper J (ed) Occupational therapy in oncology and palliative care. Wiley, London, p 176

Bray J, Cooper J 2005 The contribution to palliative medicine of allied health professions – the contribution of occupational therapy. In: Doyle D, Hanks G, Cherny N, Calman K (eds) Oxford textbook of palliative medicine, 3rd edn. Oxford University Press, Oxford, p 135

Bye R 1998 When clients are dying: occupational therapists' perspectives. Occupational Therapy Journal of Research 18(1):3–24

Cherny N I 2004 The problem of suffering. In: Doyle D, Hanks G, Cherny N, Calman K (eds) Oxford textbook of palliative medicine, 3rd edn. Oxford University Press, Oxford, pp 7–14

Cheville A L 2000 Cancer rehabilitation and palliative care. In: Rehabilitation in oncology. Online. Available: http://findarticles.com/p/articles 7 Sept 2006

Chochinov H, Wilson K, Enns M et al 1997 Are you depressed? Screening for depression in the terminally ill. American Journal of Psychiatry 154(5):674–676

Cooper J 2005 Occupational therapy in oncology and palliative care. Wiley, London, pp 11–25

Cooper J, Littlechild B 2004 A study of occupational therapy interventions in oncology and palliative care. International Journal of Therapy and Rehabilitation 11(7):329–334

Doyle D 2005 Foreword. In: Cooper J (ed) Occupational therapy in oncology and palliative care. Wiley, Chichester, p xii

Horne R 2005 Self care. Presentation at: Enhancing self care – the evidence base. 3–5 May, Alliance for Self Care Research Conference, Dundee

Hotopf M, Chidgey J, Addington-Hall J et al 2002 Depression in advanced disease: Part 1 Prevalence and case-finding. Palliative Medicine 16:81–97

Hynson J L, Sawyer S M 2001 Paediatric palliative care: distinctive needs and emerging issues. Journal of Paediatric Child Health 37:323–325

Krishnasamy M 1997 Exploring the nature and impact of fatigue in cancer. International Journal of Palliative Nursing 3(3):126–131

Kubler-Ross E 1983 On children and death. Macmillan, New York, p 24

Lowrie D 2006 Occupational therapy and cancer-related fatigue. In: Cooper J (ed) Occupational therapy in oncology and palliative care. London, Wiley, pp 61–81

McCluskey U 2005 To be met as a person. Karnac, London

Randall F, Downie R S 1999 Palliative care ethics – a companion for all specialties. Oxford University Press, Oxford

Royal College of Paediatrics and Child Health (1997) Prevention and control of pain in children – a manual for health care professionals. British Medical Journal Publications, London

Saunders C 1993 Foreword. In: Doyle D, Hanks G W C, MacDonald N (eds) Oxford textbook of palliative medicine. Oxford University Press, Oxford

Siegel B 1999 Love, medicine and miracles. Random House, London

Stone P 2002 The measurement, causes and effective management of cancer related fatigue. International Journal of Palliative Nursing 8(3):120–128

Symington J 2000 Imprisoned pain and its transformation. Karnac, London

Twycross A 1998 Dispelling modern day myths about children's pain. Journal of Child Health Care 2(1): 31–35

Weininger O 1996 Being and not being – clinical applications of the death instinct. Karnac, London, p 135

Winnicott D W 1964 The child, the family, and the outside world. Penguin, London, p 170

World Health Organization 1998 Cancer pain relief and palliative care in children. WHO, Geneva

Suggested further reading

Edmonton Staging System 2006 Assessment tools. In: Edmonton Palliative Care programme. Online. Available: http://www.palliative.org 9 Sept 2006

Firth S 2001 Wider horizons – care of the dying in a multicultural society. National Council for Hospice and Specialist Care Services, London. Online. Available: http://www.hospice-spc-council. org.uk 4 May 2006

National Council for Palliative Care & Department of Health 2006 Introductory guide to end of life care in care homes. Online. Available: http://www.endoflifecare.nhs.uk 4 May 2006

NHS Scotland 2002 Clinical standards – specialist palliative care. Clinical Standards Board for Scotland, Edinburgh. Online. Available: http://www.clinicalstandards.org 5 Aug 2006

Morgan G 2000 Assessment of quality of life in palliative care. International Journal of Palliative Nursing 6(8):406–410

Appendix 4.1
Pain assessment in children

Claire Tester

'By any reasonable code, freedom from pain should be a basic human right, limited only by our knowledge to achieve it', wrote Liebeskind & Melzack (1988). But pain is still undiagnosed in infants and young children, and for people who cannot communicate and may have a developmental delay. Existing pain assessment tools focus on physical pain, and are for children who are cognitively aware, able to communicate their pain, and have a concept of the degree of pain. For children aged 3 years and up, the Faces Scale (Wong & Baker 1988) and the Oucher (Huff & Joshi 2001) both require children to identify their pain with either a cartoon or photograph of a face showing pain, whereas pain is colour coded in Eland's Color Tool (McConahay et al 2006) and the Poker Chip Tool (Huff & Joshi 2001). There are two scales for infants and toddlers; the Objective Pain Scale and the CRIES (Huff & Joshi 2001), which both rely on behavioural and physiological measures. These are all scales to assess the degree of analgesia required but it is difficult to differentiate an infant's emotional distress from physical pain. For example, children can become distressed and upset, experiencing a real sense of loss of the familiar as they enter the hospice or hospital environment. It is the mother or main caregiver who can soothe and calm the child. When mother is not present the child experiences a further deeper loss (Bowlby 1997). Such distress can presents as the child in pain, but it is emotional, not physical. Physical symptoms such as headache or stomach ache can present if the emotional distress is not resolved (see Ch. 3). As part of pain and symptom assessment it is necessary to have information at first hand on the behaviour of the child when distressed and how that child can be reassured and soothed. This may be with a cuddle, a favourite toy, a favourite blanket to hold, etc.

References

Bowlby J 1997 Attachment and loss, 2nd edn. Pimlico, London, vol 1

Huff S, Joshi P 2001 Pain and symptom management. In: Armstrong-Dailey A, Zarbock S (eds) Hospice care for children. Oxford University Press, Oxford

Liebeskind J C, Melzack R 1988 The International Pain Foundation: meeting a need for education in pain management. Journal of Pain Symptom Management. 3(3):131–132

McConahay T, Bryson M, Bulloch B 2006 Defining mild, moderate, and severe pain by using the color analog scale with children presenting to a pediatric emergency department. Academic Emergency Medicine Journal 13(3):341–344. Online. Available: http://www.aemj.org 1 Dec 2006

Wong D, Baker C 1988 Pain in children: a comparison of assessment scales. Pediatric Nursing 14(1):9–17

Appendix 4.2
Children's care plans

Claire Tester
Background to care planning

Since the introduction of the 1989 Children Act (England) there has been a duty to assess the needs and services for children who were sick and/or disabled and deemed 'children in need' (ACT et al 2001). This Act for children was developed from the Chronically Sick and Disabled Persons Act 1970. In 1996 it was a requirement that local registers of children were kept with a disability and the needs of these children were identified in Joint Children's Service Plans. However, it was felt that children with life-limiting conditions or who were terminally ill and with complex needs were not recognised and included. This led to the report, 'Guide to the Development of Children's Palliative Care Services', produced by the Association for Children with Life-Threatening or Terminal Conditions and Their Families (ACT 1997) recommending flexible care plans.

The guidance produced for professionals in 2000 under the title 'Framework for the Assessment of Children in Need and their Families' related to vulnerable children, but again did not relate to the palliative care needs of children (DoH et al 2000). In 1997 ACT published 'Guide to the Development of Children's Palliative Care Services' for both professionals and families.

The more recent (2003) 'Guide to Effective Care Planning – Assessment of Children with Life-limiting Conditions and Their Families' encourages a wide range of assessment of needs and coordination of services and support for the child, young person and family.

The summary of needs includes:

- personal care – including ADL
- symptom management – control and relief of symptoms
- symptom management – using therapies
- aids and equipment
- respite care
- psychological and emotional support
- spiritual support
- financial needs
- education.

Additional needs for young people are:

- transition to adult clinical services, adult social services, and independent living
- college/university
- employment
- sexual needs.

An overview

These care plans are to ensure the quality of palliative care and therapy. They are primarily for the *child*, to consider all the needs of the child, emotional and psychological, developmental as well as physical. All care plans should be accurate, up to date, meaningful and relevant to the child or young person.

The key points for writing care plans are:

1. Foremost for the child or young person, who can be actively involved in making the plan.
2. For parents and families: to assure that their child's needs are understood and that the parents can develop a confidence and trust in the staff that their child will be looked after in the way they would wish. This includes cultural and religious considerations.
3. For the staff: to do their job to the best of their ability.
4. To be shared with other staff in other settings for continuity of care, e.g. hospital, respite.
5. To ensure standards of care are met.
6. To be understood. Parents, staff and carers will read the plans, so the language should be clear and jargon free. Young people should have access to their own plans, which they can review, and change with staff.
7. To be coordinated with services. There may be a number of different care plans made: at school; in hospital, hospice, and respite home; and by community staff for the child at home. This would seem a lot of duplication, and it is the child or young person who experiences the differences and any disparity of approach. Ideally it would be helpful to have a single shared plan.

Completing the care plan is usually the task of the key worker but should involve everyone who is involved. This can be a helpful exercise in itself if there is a large number of health professionals involved with the child directly. It provides an opportunity to consider the experience of the child and how the way in which practitioners work might be reconfigured, for example providing advice and training to the parents and key worker directly.

References

ACT Association for Children with Life-threatening or Terminal Conditions and their Families 1993 (revised 1998) ACT Charter for Children with Life Threatening Conditions and their Families. ACT, Bristol

ACT Association for Children with Life-threatening or Terminal Conditions and their Families 1997 Guide to the development of children's palliative care services. ACT, Bristol

ACT Association for Children with Life-threatening or Terminal Conditions and their Families 2003 A Guide to effective care planning – assessment of children with life limiting conditions and their families. ACT, Bristol. Online. Available: http://www.act.org.uk 25 Oct 2006

Association for Children with Life-threatening or Terminal Conditions and their Families/National Council for Hospice and Specialist Palliative Care Services/Scottish Partnership Agency for Palliative and Cancer Care 2001 Palliative care for young people 13–24. ACT, Bristol. Online. Available: http://www.act.org.uk 10 Sept 2006

Children Act 1989. HMSO, London

Chronically Sick and Disabled Persons Act 1970. HMSO, London

Department of Health, Department for Education and Employment and The Home Office 2000 The framework for the assessment of children in need and their families. The Stationery Office, London

Appendix 4.3
Home from Home comfort map

Claire Tester

A child's confusion, anxiety and pain can be exacerbated by disorientation and being in a strange environment and bed on a hospital ward. Hospital procedures and a change of staff on a shift pattern all contribute. The parents' own anxiety in this new and unfamiliar situation and their own sense of vulnerability and powerlessness to change the situation can contribute to the child's anxiety. Existing pain assessments address physical pain but there are different types of pain which have an emotional basis and cannot be physically located, or controlled by medication. Anxiety and fear are experienced as painful by children but are not usually addressed as part of pain management. Emotional pain needs to be understood. In applying ethical principles it is necessary to identify and provide support for the child. This is different from the support parents and siblings require. Each child is an individual with a unique framework for support, reassurance and comfort. It is not enough to intuit or guess (Ward & McMahon 1998).

Home from Home map (Tester 2005, unpublished work)

The intention is to create a cocoon of safety and familiarity for the infant or child, a familiarity for the child in the child's own space. In this way the child may feel comforted and reassured. It is necessary to identify the child's own individual framework, and the comfort map and its picture format is a way of doing this. The Home from Home comfort map is a worksheet to record information on what reassures the child. This map is intended for infants and young children but could be adapted for young adults and adults as appropriate. It is for use in a hospital or hospice environment, although its use is not limited to palliative care. It is to be compiled with parents in an interview with staff before the child's admission to a hospital or hospice. The child may actively contribute, depending upon age and ability.

It is necessary to know what reassures the child in the absence of the main caregiver. Sleeping and settling routines always incorporate something familiar and the same. This is often overlooked because, although parents do have their own bedtime rituals for their child, they may not be recognised as such. For example, a mobile the child fixes upon before sleep, a particular tune played on a musical box or toy, and the bedding itself such as a sheepskin or a blanket. Parents may have a small picture bedside light with moving images. One particular special toy which is always placed near the child is comforting, usually a soft toy which can be held. Very large and giant soft toys are room ornaments rather than comforters.

Small children may have a familiar routine together with a story. For toddlers this is often the same story read over again each night in the same way. For some children an item belonging to their mother is held and kept, and can accompany the child during the day, such as a scarf which may have the mother's perfume scent, if she wears one. Tapes can be made of stories read by a parent who reads the stories at home. The story book can be taken from home with the child and held open with a member of staff as the tape is played.

The move into the hospital or hospice can be in itself such a big experience for the family, regardless of length of stay, that small things can be overlooked. There is also the idea that these things may be lost. They need to be named, or even an identical toy or object purchased and introduced at home, washed for the right smell and 'softening' period.

At a children's hospice there is a sensitivity to creating a welcoming room for the child. Over time the same things can be used in the room, e.g. same patterned duvet cover, a mobile, soft toys and pictures, but initially these are all strange and familiarity builds up over time.

Information to include on the map

a. The child's name.

b. The child's comforter – e.g. specific toy or object such as special blanket.

c. Special cup, or teat and bottle.

d. Positioning in being held, sleeping position. This is particularly important for children with extensor or flexor spasms and contractures.

e. Comforting sounds such as heartbeat sounds, special songs.

f. Things enjoyed: activities, food and drink, comforting smells, massage, etc.

g. The signs and behaviour indicating discomfort, pain and distress.

h. What upsets, unsettles the child. What the child does not like. This should include sounds, approaches, toys, positioning, activities, as well as food and drinks.

i. A list of things to bring in, such as toy, photographs, books, tapes/CDs, quilt or blanket, any games, etc. Each of these should be named and checked against this list on arrival, during the stay, and at the end of the stay. It is helpful to save these items in a special box or bag which is near to hand.

j. The names of siblings, pets, grandparents, e.g. Nan, as well as relevant names of important people in the child's life. Such information can help staff talk to the child about the child's family and encourage a sharing and discussion.

This list is not exhaustive and the parents of the child may suggest other aspects that are not included here. It has been found helpful for parents to have discussions with staff who are concerned and interested in how to comfort their child, and how to reassure the child in ways that are familiar. As one parent remarked, 'I really felt the staff wanted to do what we did as parents, and to get it right. I felt so reassured.'

The Home from Home comfort map is a pictorial worksheet which is to be openly displayed rather than filed. In this way it is visible and accessible to staff as it is near the child.

Reference

Ward A, McMahon L 1998 Intuition is not enough. Routledge, London

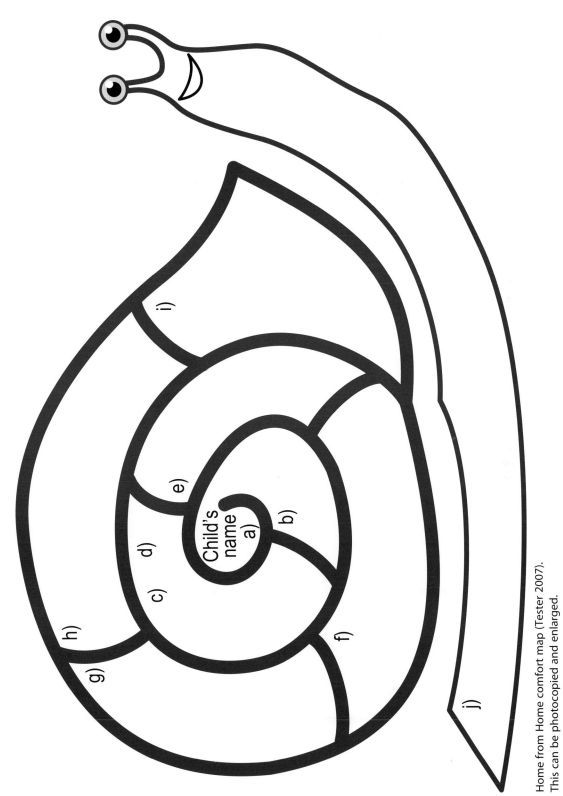

Child's name

a)
b)
c)
d)
e)
f)
g)
h)
i)
j)

Home from Home comfort map (Tester 2007).
This can be photocopied and enlarged.

Spirituality

Kathryn Boog

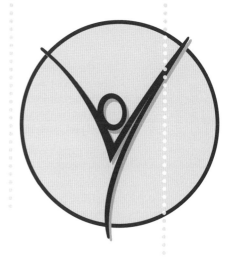

Our deeds travel with us from afar,
And what we have been makes us what we are.

George Eliot

Key words

meaning; challenges; communication; creativity; culture; pain; hope

5

The highly subjective and intangible nature of spirituality makes it difficult to define. Its components can be elusive, shrouded in that ethereal and indefinable quality attributed to dreams and musings, and yet they are as real to the individual who experiences them as the objects, events and people that they embody. Individuals' beliefs about themselves and their relationships to the people and things that surround and influence them, and that they influence, will provide the bedrock of their lives. They are something against which people gauge their experiences and base their plans, with cultural influences playing a large part in spiritual identity, shaping and moulding the core components that make us who we are.

Many people find their identity and confirm their status through the things that they do, such as their job, their role (Saunders 1998) or their leisure activities (McGrath 2002). Whilst able to continue with these occupations, they may not have given much consideration to the deeper meanings associated with their lives, and how these have influenced their life's journey.

An event that challenges people's image of themselves can, however, shake these deeply rooted beliefs and precipitate feelings of insecurity as they view their situation as lurching out of control. They need to reconnect with their previous values in order to regain their sense of self and re-establish their status and worth.

The prospect of imminent death can trigger a change in people's values and a shift in focus from the material aspects of their lives to the spiritual, promoting a need to consolidate connections with the things that matter most. What are their passions, what drives them, what gives them a buzz and makes their hearts sing? What gives them comfort and holds them firm, rooting them in their past, present and future?

In today's society, people's spiritual orientations are wide-ranging and may be drawn not only from a broad array of religious beliefs, but also include complementary and alternative approaches, such as New Age philosophies. These eclectic views will be reflected in conversation and choice of activity, both of these providing useful clues to who a person is, and what that person needs, offering guidance towards ensuring suitable and timely intervention for those with existential concerns (Hunt 2003). Spirituality, then, is best viewed as the 'I' in living and dying.

Professionals' own spirituality

In order to recognise the spiritual element in someone else, healthcare professionals need first of all to consider their own standpoint, to identify their own values and beliefs and reflect on how these guide their lives and their practice (Belcham 2004). Self-awareness will be an advantage in identifying the reasons behind any difficult emotions experienced by health professionals, and in helping find ways to deal with these (Stolick 2003), whilst being in tune with their own spirituality will make it easier to recognise in others.

In striving to attain professional credibility, healthcare workers have identified with the medical model and in recent years have ignored the intangible and elusive components of spiritual care. The modern-day approach recognises the need to encompass the whole spectrum of needs in order to provide effective care, and that includes spiritual and existential issues. For health professionals, it is not enough to merely acknowledge this requisite for holistic care. They will only be able to assist the patient to achieve spiritual well-being if they have an awareness of its importance (Collins 2006) and can direct patients to the appropriate person in the multidisciplinary team to help with the issues, if they find that they are unable to do this themselves (Walter 1997).

Defining spirituality is like catching a cloud

Much time and effort in the past has been spent in the pursuit of a definition for spirituality, and its relationship to religion. The modern approach, however, suggests that rather than search for an all-encompassing definition on which to base their approach, health professionals should support patients in the discovery of the significance of their own unique experiences (Stanworth 2002) and the personal values that are bestowed on these during the individual's spiritual journey (Collins 2006). People can be oblivious to this spiritual element to their lives, and when they realise its existence, can be surprised at how much this enhances their quality of life.

Jim felt he had failed in everything he had tried in life – education (he had a very poor reading ability), work (he had been unable to remain in any job for longer than 3 months) and relationships (three failed marriages by the age of 40) and now his health. The discovery of an undiscovered and incredibly creative ability in painting demonstrated at last a facet of himself that he would not have believed possible, and meant that, in his last few weeks of life, he was able at last to realise his potential, to find status and credibility and to leave behind gifts that he felt were worthy of the people closest to him.

Individuals need to be supported in this quest for meaning and enlightenment, but not directed towards another's idea of what this might be (Frankl 1987). They need to regain control over the things that they hold dear, re-establishing a sense of self and reinstating their purpose in life.

This abstract nature of spirituality is what makes it difficult for individuals to explain and define. For those from a religious background, relating to the traditions and rituals and using the accepted language of their particular faith, will make sharing their beliefs easier.

> Sarah found great comfort in certain pictures that were connected to her religious beliefs. She was aware of her family's struggles to accept her illness and felt that sharing copies of these pictures with them might be helpful. The originals were scanned, and Sarah mounted copies in small frames with messages to each person put on the back.

For others, explaining this very personal, diverse and subjective facet of their personality may be much more complex and, indeed, they may not find it possible to describe it in words. In this instance, making a connection, perhaps through health professional and patient working together in a companionable silence, may allow for the introduction of alternative ways to identify and work through areas of spiritual importance. By adopting a creative approach, perhaps through the use of art or crafts or memory album work, it is possible for people to find an acceptable way to express that internal being (Egan & deLaat 1994).

65

> Dave's family were so important to him. He had spent much of their early lives working away from home, providing the finance for their education and exotic family holidays. He had precious memories of his sons as small children, of things they had done together, and some of their funny, child-like conversations. He wondered if they remembered too? It concerned him that they might just have memories of an absent father and he felt he had to let them know how much he had treasured reminiscing over these stories in his lonely hotel rooms across the world. He worked on a memory album for them, in 5- to 10-minute stretches, and special photos were scanned in. Together, the family laughed and reminisced over the stories and shared others, revealing all their love for their father despite his concerns.

Patients will choose for themselves who they want to confide in, and listening to their stories (Stolick 2003, Walter 1997) will help to determine an understanding of what spirituality means to each specific person, providing the basis for supporting that person's particular needs. By focusing on patients' own lives and drawing attention to the things that they feel passionate about, health professionals can help people to find their direction, and to continue with their own spiritual journey.

In view of the lack of research into cross-cultural issues relating to existential distress (Blinderman & Cherny 2005), this approach, listening to the narratives of patient and family (Chiang & Carlson 2003) and knowing enough of their cultural background to ask questions

(Cheraghi et al 2005) will assist the health professional to glean the elements that will contribute to good spiritual care.

Offering a presence, just being there (Lugton 2002) and giving time and attention, and acknowledging the stories that are meaningful to the individual will give credence to people's lives and make them feel worthy and valued. Counselling skills will be useful here, where the non-judgmental approach used, alongside an acceptance of that person's beliefs and values, will encourage disclosure. There will always be some common ground for conversation, and making this link with someone will help in the development of a supportive relationship.

Spiritual pain

When people are reviewing their lives, an inability to find meaning and purpose – their raison d'être – may result in spiritual or soul pain (Rahman 2000) and feelings of regret that their lives have not turned out the way that they would have hoped (Walter 2002). These may relate to a sense of lost opportunities, or be the result of conflict within relationships. Poor communication can be further exacerbated by patients' reluctance to share existential issues with families and carers for fear of adding to their burdens, or of embarrassing themselves and those closest to them (Searle et al 2000). The family's response may be to withdraw from the situation, sometimes to the extent of acting as if the person is no longer a family member, thereby adding to the spiritual distress (Saunders 1988).

'The spectre of death reveals our relationships to be our most precious possessions' (Byock 2004) and is possibly the reason that so many people seek closeness, reconciliation and forgiveness from others at this time. The nearness of death uncovers issues that have remained hidden and unresolved for years 'because nothing can remain hidden when there's so little time left, and when everything that was acting as a screen suddenly looks so flimsy' (de Hennezel 1997).

People still hope that they will be able to achieve certain things before they die, and the realisation that they will not be able to participate in future events within the family, such as seeing their children mature into adults, or growing old with a beloved partner is a further cause of spiritual anguish in the dying (McGrath 2002). People need to feel that they will be remembered, that some aspect of their being will outlive them, and that their influence might still be a part of rituals and family events in years to come.

Molly knew that her daughter might not remember her. Susie was only 2 and unaware of her mother's anguish at not being there to see her daughter grow into a woman. She decided to buy and to make, gifts for every birthday until Susie reached 16. Each was carefully chosen and created with great love and care. The presents were then wrapped and, accompanied by a hand made card for each birthday, placed in a special box with instructions to Molly's husband to present each to Susie on the appropriate birthday. Molly hoped they would let her daughter know just how much she was loved and maybe keep her real in Susie's memory.

Unacceptable changes to the physical self, resulting in concerns around how people feel about themselves and how they appear and are accepted by others can also be a determining factor in the experience of total pain, and cultural influences may be a significant factor in this respect.

Regaining a purpose in life counteracts poor self-esteem and demoralisation (Kissane et al 2001), challenging existential distress by returning meaning and a sense of satisfaction to life, and restoring dignity (Chochinov et al 2005) and self-esteem.

> Jane reflecting on meeting a new challenge: 'You need to be satisfied with what you've done. That gives you confidence and you learn from experience and build on that.'

Activities to respond to spiritual needs and encourage and facilitate spiritual expression

Because of the different meanings that individuals ascribe to the experiences of living and dying, whether these be cultural, familial, religious or secular, getting to know them as the unique persons that they are and identifying their discrete hopes, needs and goals is the only way to determine the support that they need to write the final chapter of their lives. Listening to the life narrative will indicate what matters most – perhaps making connections with others, visiting a special place one last time, enjoying the marvels of nature, continuing to participate in certain events and activities, or maintaining a role. Identifying what a person wants to do most and providing the means and the encouragement to progress with the idea, will be a stimulating and motivating experience. The maintenance of activities related to roles and status is of great importance to some people and professionals need to think creatively about how to prolong their participation in these.

> Su-lin had always loved food – buying it, preparing and cooking it and best of all, eating it. She enthused over favourite recipes and recalled stories of family gatherings when she was a child, describing the colours, textures and smells to the staff at the hospice. Despite the ravages of her progressive neurological disease, she was still able to savour the delights of her national cuisine and enjoyed sharing recipes with others.
>
> *'If I couldn't enjoy food in some way, I think I would die!'*
>
> Many people asked her for her recipes and Su-lin wanted to share her love with others and so a calendar was developed, using the computer, with recipes dictated and transcribed on to the pages. Together with the OT who acted as her hands, Su-lin made a collage, which was then scanned in as the front cover. The finished calendar was given as a gift to friends and Su-lin asked for copies to be sold in the hospice shop so that she could give something back for the care she had enjoyed.

Participation in activities that connect to the spirit allows individuals to experience 'flow' (Csikszentmihalyi 1990) – to lose themselves in the moment, to be in touch with their secret, inner self and provide an outlet for the associated feelings.

> James, on his participation in silk painting: 'You've really got to concentrate – you get away into yourself and it's as if you're on your own although you're in a crowd.'

67

People will choose to participate in activities that reflect their spiritual needs (Engquist et al 1996) and should be given the opportunity to reconnect with past activities that gave their life meaning, albeit they may need to pursue these in a modified way. The accomplishment of precious activities will produce positive, pleasurable feelings for both the patient and the facilitator, nurturing the spirit and fostering hope, whilst mastering new ones may result in the discovery of inner strengths and surprise at the pleasure gained in the achievement of activities that the person had not considered previously, or thought were impossible.

> Ann, talking about glass painting: 'Doing these things gives me a challenge – working out colours, where I will hang the finished mirror, things like that.'

The diversity of individual personalities and the spiritual influences on these are described in the following examples.

Equipment provision

As the ability to care for themselves diminishes, people are more able to accept their limitations if independence in even small areas can be maintained. A creative approach is useful here, using careful forward planning and pre-empting deterioration, and the gradual replacement of unachievable goals with more attainable, but still acceptable ones. These, alongside positioning and the provision of assistive equipment for activities of daily living and leisure pursuits, will allow for continuing participation for as long as the patient wants.

> Michael needed to have everything done for him. He had no energy and was breathless and pained when he moved. He felt that slight movements in his position helped, but did not want to be constantly calling the nurses, despite their assurances that it was not a problem. Michael wanted to be able to control the adjustments to his bed by himself, but couldn't reach the control. To do this independently would mean he would not be impatient and restless whilst trying not to call for help. The OT gave him a small piece of equipment, produced from a piece of dowel and a rubber thimble that allowed him to operate the controls of his bed – he was delighted and able now to relax.

Body image

How they look, and dealing with hygiene and grooming, can be very important to some people, even those very close to death. They may need help to maintain independence in this, as in other aspects of their lives, and beauty therapy, including make-up, wigs, scarves, manicures and complementary therapies can all enhance their feelings about their body image and how others see them. This may be of particular importance where people are unable to do anything for themselves and will enhance feeling of self-worth, boosting their self-esteem at a time when it is low.

> Anna had been given a prosthesis several years ago following her mastectomy. She had never worn it and it was now lost. During a dressing practice, she hinted that she wished she had it to wear now, as she felt lop-sided and self-conscious now that friends and colleagues were seeing her in her nightwear. The therapist ordered a new one for her, and Anna remarked that she felt like a new woman, and wished she had worn the prosthesis years ago and that she now had the confidence to see old friends and colleagues who she had been turning away.

Being remembered for the person that they are or were

People have their own impressions of themselves and how they appear to others. For some, how they have been in the past is of great importance and they want to convey a flavour of what they consider to be their real selves to new acquaintances, such as health professionals and the other people attending day care. Bringing things to day hospice to share with others is an example of this. Bakers bring cakes; gardeners bring plants, e.g. flowers and tomatoes; some bring photographs of themselves with friends and family. Inpatients may enjoy making a collage of themselves before they were ill, to hang in their room, whilst people with communication difficulties may like to help produce a journal that displays the things that are important for others to know about them.

> Rob had spent many years raising funds for charity. He had walked the length and breadth of Scotland, wearing the kilt and accompanied by his dog Smudge. He wanted people to remember him as the broad, strapping man he had been then instead of the emaciated shadow of himself. Using a photo of Rob and his dog, taken on one of his walks, the therapist worked with him to make cards for his friends, scanning the picture on to the front and adding humorous captions. Inside, he wrote his last messages for them.

Others want to ensure that they will be remembered in the way that they would have liked (Rahman 2000). Memory albums and boxes allow people to tell their stories the way they want them to be, and for dying parents who want the hospice experience to be remembered in a positive way by their child, activities that can be shared should be encouraged.

Gift and card making and letter writing are all methods used in memory making, as are videos, CDs and tapes, both visual and audio, consisting of words and particular songs and pieces of music. These are used in some funeral services and may be included in a printed order of service.

Creativity

For people attempting to seek out and identify the spiritual element of their personality, the opportunity to participate in creative activities can provide the key. This newly acquired knowledge can then be used to advantage, allowing people to give vent to their feelings and their innermost thoughts and nurturing the soul through allowing it a means of expression (Burkhardt & Nagai-Jacobson 1994).

> Clare, talking about making gifts for her family and friends: 'When I'm making things, it's very personal to me. I feel that I'm putting a little bit of myself into everything I do.'

Unfinished business and closure

This may relate to relationships and the reinstating of lost connections, as discussed at length in Chapter 12. It may also involve decision making about who will inherit what. Patients may want to wrap small items and write cards and letters to accompany them. People may want to organise their finances or arrange their funeral, not just the service, but what they want to be dressed in, and what others should wear and how they want their life celebrated.

Linking with nature

In guided imagery, people will choose a time and a place that has deep meaning for them, and by visualising that whole experience, recreate the feelings of joy and contentment that they had at that time. This often involves their involvement with a natural phenomenon and the senses that were stimulated at that time, such as the relaxing sound of waves on a beach, the crunch of crisp autumn leaves underfoot, a beautiful tropical sunset, the smell of a new baby. Similarly, tending

69

to plants, nurturing them and watching them grow allows people to create something that will live on beyond them and be enjoyed by others in the future.

Hope

People's hopes and aspirations are linked to the spiritual side of their nature. Fostering hope means addressing their spiritual needs – looking at the whole picture and listening to their inner voice in order to direct them along a path towards the fulfilment of precious goals. With the achievement of these needs and dreams, the spiritual element of existence can be nurtured and savoured, allowing patients to complete that final stage of their life's journey knowing that they have done their best, and offering hope for a future they will not see.

Thinking of children and young people

Spirituality is not usually considered as part of the thinking of children and adolescents, perceived as only experienced by adults, but this is wrong as there is sense of leaving a life behind, and of wondering where they are going. As one child aged 10 years asked, 'Will my family remember me? How?' Such questions should be gently and sensitively explored at the child's pace, taking care not to assume what the child is saying, nor to conflict with strongly held beliefs if they are helpful to the child or young person. This can also lead to developing ideas for activities and keepsakes the child or young person wishes to leave. It can also lead to a discussion about a living will. As one young adult said, 'My brother can have my old Celtic top but I want to keep the new one.'

Depending upon age, a child may have a sense of spirituality closely linked with religious ideas and belief. Children ask about heaven and about God, their understanding reliant upon what they have been told by family, and school. They fill in the gaps in their knowledge with imagination.

> 8-year-old boy whose 5-year-old sister is terminally ill: 'I think God will let down an invisible magic rope ladder for my sister to climb up to heaven soon.'

Religious education may be the only information a child may have about the end of life, and all that has been heard and read is recalled and questioned. Children hear about hell too and imagination fills in the horror. It is necessary to ascertain what the family believe and reinforce it, although the information can be difficult to obtain when a child feels you are to be trusted to give an honest and open answer on the spot.

> 14-year-old adolescent boy asking occupational therapist: 'What is heaven like?'
>
> Occupational therapist: 'Well, that's a good question because we would all like to know. The difficult thing is that no one has come back and told everyone all about it. I think everyone has ideas though, which are always very good. What do you think?'

This question led to a long discussion about anxieties and fear, which required careful counselling by the therapist, who then introduced the idea of exploring some of these ideas with the chaplain. For young people adolescence is a time of struggling with an emerging identity and existential thoughts. Discussions can be philosophical as young adults struggle to understand what is happening to them, and try to understand why. For some adolescents the idea of discussing such things with a chaplain or priest can be difficult, for as one 17-year-old man remarked, 'Well I know what he's going to say, and I don't think I agree with all that dogma.'

When a child or young person dies in a hospice or on a hospital ward, this impacts upon others in the environment and can throw them into further questioning of spirituality, of meaning and purpose in life, and death.

'He was the same age as me. He had what I've got,' said an 18-year-old young woman.

Staff can understandably find it difficult to explain, but a willingness to listen, to support, and to not know with a young person is better than ignoring and walking by.

Chapters 3 and 6 offer some further insight. Also see Appendix 12.4 on therapeutic communication with children.

References

Belcham C 2004 Spirituality in occupational therapy: theory in practice? British Journal of Occupational Therapy 67(1):39–46

Blinderman C D, Cherny N I 2005 Existential issues do not necessarily result in existential suffering: lessons from cancer patients in Israel. Palliative Medicine 19:371–380

Burkhardt M, Nagai-Jacobson M G 1994 Reawakening spirit in clinical practice. Journal of Holistic Nursing 12(1):9–21

Byock I 2004 The four things that matter most. Free Press, New York, p 4

Cheraghi M A, Payne S, Salsali M 2005 Spiritual aspects of end-of-life care for Muslim patients: experiences from Iran. International Journal of Palliative Nursing 11(9):468–474

Chiang M, Carlson G 2003 Occupational therapy in multicultural contexts: issues and strategies. British Journal of Occupational Therapy 66(12):559–567

Chochinov H, Hack T, Hassard T et al 2005 Dignity therapy: a novel psychotherapeutic intervention for patients near the end of life. Journal of Clinical Oncology 23(24):5520–5525

Collins M 2006 Unfolding spirituality: working with and beyond definitions. International Journal of Therapy and Rehabilitation 13(6):254–257

Csikszentmihalyi M 1990 Flow: the psychology of optimal experience. Harper and Row, New York

de Hennezel M 1997 Intimate death: how the dying teach us to live. Warner, London

Egan M, deLaat M D 1994 Considering spirituality in occupational therapy practice. Canadian Journal of Occupational Therapy 61(2):95–101

Engquist D E, Short-DeGraff M, Gliner J et al 1996 Occupational therapists' beliefs and practices with regard to spirituality and therapy. American Journal of Occupational Therapy 51(3):173–180

Frankl V E 1987 Man's search for meaning. Revised and enlarged edn. Hodder and Stoughton, London

Hunt J 2003 The quality of spiritual care – developing a standard. International Journal of Palliative Nursing 9(5):208–215

Kissane D W, Clarke DM, Street AF 2001 Demoralization syndrome – a relevant psychiatric diagnosis for palliative care. Journal of Palliative Care 17(1):12–21

Lugton J 2002 Communicating with dying people and their relatives. Radcliffe Medical Press, Oxford

McGrath P 2002 New horizons in spirituality research. In: Rumbold B (ed) Spirituality in palliative care. Oxford University Press, Oxford, pp 178–194

Rahman H 2000 Journey of providing care in hospice: perspectives of occupational therapists. Qualitative Health Research 10(6):806–818

Saunders C 1988 Spiritual pain. Journal of Palliative Care 4(3):29–32

Searle C, Finlay I, Owen N 2000 Spiritual needs: use of focus groups to identify and address spiritual pain. Palliative Care Today 52–54

Stanworth R 2002 Attention: a potential vehicle for spiritual care. Journal of Palliative Care 18(3):192–195

Stolick M 2003 Dying to meet you: facing mortality and enabling patient styles. American Journal of Hospice and Palliative Care 20(4):269–273

Walter T 1997 The ideology and organisation of spiritual care: three approaches. Palliative Medicine 11:21–30

Walter T 2002 Spirituality in palliative care: opportunity or burden? Palliative Medicine 16:133–139

Bereavement – the pain of loving

Claire Tester

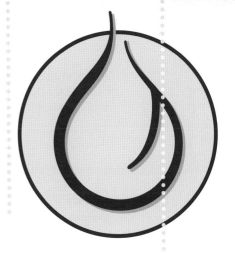

'Begin at the beginning', the King said gravely, 'and go on till you come to the end: then stop.'

Lewis Carroll

Key words

bereavement: anticipatory grief; mourning; loss

6

Introduction

Bereavement is the loss of a relationship or love of someone, or something. It is usually associated with the death of a loved one, but mourning and grief can begin before death, and can be experienced by the person who is dying. An overview of the current thinking on bereavement, together with considerations on loss as experienced by the living, of themselves, and of anticipatory bereavement will be discussed. Definitions (Thesaurus 2006) of words used to describe bereavement and aspects associated with it are given below.

Bereavement; *Definition:* **loss**
Synonyms: affliction, deprivation, distress, misfortune, sorrow

Grief; *Definition:* **suffering**
Synonyms: agony, anguish, bereavement, dejection, depression, desolation, despair, despondency, discomfort, disquiet, distress, gloom, grievance, melancholy, misery, pain, regret, sadness, sorrow, suffering, torture, trial, unhappiness, worry, wretchedness

Loss; *Definition:* **misfortune**
Synonyms: accident, bad luck, bereavement, catastrophe, damage, defeat, deficiency, deprivation, destruction, disappearance, disaster, failure, impairment, injury, ruin, sacrifice, trial, trouble, want, waste, wreckage

Mourning; *Definition:* **sadness**

Synonyms: aching, bereavement, crying, grief, grieving, languishing, moaning, pining, sorrowing, wailing, weeping, woe

These definitions and synonyms indicate the depth and range of the deep emotional pain and trauma of bereavement, which will now be explored.

Overview

As each of us grows older, life can be viewed as a series of changes each of which involves loss, for to embrace a new or different situation is to leave another behind. Some losses are relatively small, such as leaving school or moving house; others such as the diagnosis of a life-limiting incurable condition involve the loss of one's perceived future and sense of that future self; but the loss of a loved person who has died can plunge the bereaved into an all-encompassing grief. All losses, regardless of magnitude involve resistance, acceptance and readjustment to living in a different situation. But the more profound the loss, the more severe and painful is the experience, and the longer it takes to accept the loss. In 1917 Freud (1991) recognised that mourning regularly accompanied 'the loss of a loved person, or loss of some abstraction . . . such as one's country, liberty, and ideal or so on'. Freud perceived the loss of a loved person or object as a loss of a part of the self. This leaves the person living with a break or hole in the psyche, as if a part were missing. This is reinforced in everyday language when married people describe their spouse as their 'other half'.

Bereavement is understood to be something to recover from (Guntrip 1992), and a normal process which can affect everyone. Whether it is understood to be a series of stages, an emotional state, a process, or a set of strategies and behaviour is dependent upon the different theoretical models. Bereavement is seen as a linear process moving from an intensely distressing experience, to a gradual acknowledgement and acceptance of the loss. People experiencing a bereavement may even describe themselves over time, as 'moving on'.

Freud's view was that it was the loss of an aspect of oneself which was linked to the past, the present and the future and internalised, for which a person grieved. He identified that there was an emerging out of a sorrowful state over time. Freud's psychoanalytical stance was that a part of the living person, or abstract lost, had to be reclaimed from the lost person (or object) as it was a part of the self, the person experiencing loss. This was the process of bereavement. This theory encouraged a belief that the living must accommodate the deceased person (or abstract aspect) as being in the past in order to live more fully in the present and to plan for the future. In this way the idea of forgetting at some level was fostered.

Parkes (1972) identified four phases within bereavement: disbelief, active searching and anger, moving to despair, followed by adjustment and acceptance. These are akin to Bowlby's attachment theory, borne out of observing the separation of young children from their mothers. Attachment theory is not a bereavement theory but is a model for loss and separation, both aspects of bereavement. Parkes' work observed aspects of attachment theory in bereavement. His model has been criticised for being a medical model with a defined process (Greenstreet 2004), with a 'problem' of suffering requiring a recovery process. However, although Parkes' stages of behaviour can be identified, they do not always follow an order, nor are they clear-cut stages. He enforces Freud's idea of moving on and letting go of a relationship which can no longer be sustained in life.

Walter (1996) proposed a new model of moving forward through the process of bereavement by not leaving the deceased behind, but rethinking and making sense of the person's life through a biography. After this task, the lost relationship is reabsorbed into the present. Walter maintained that both the relationship and the physical being of the deceased had contributed to the emotional being of the bereaved person. Neither of these could be dismissed, nor forgotten. They were part of the internal world of the bereaved person. As an extension of Walter's theory, Martin & Doka (2000) considered the effect of personality, coping strategies and gender in grieving, all creating different patterns and behaviours, and all normal. Stroebe & Schut (1999) developed a dynamic model of loss-orientated and restoration-orientated tasks involving oscillation between different states, acknowledging that the bereaved individual is not emotionally static. Restoration-orientated activities continue in parallel involving cognitive thinking such as organising the funeral, when simultaneously the bereaved person is still in disbelief (loss-orientated). This model also allows for movement backwards to an earlier experience in bereavement. There is no set pattern and there is an understanding that the pace of movement and direction of travel whether forwards or backwards is set by the individual. It is now understood that bereavement is different for everyone. The previous bereavement and loss experiences of an individual impact on the present experience of bereavement, as well as the kind of death the loved one had (Bailley et al 1999, Harwood et al 2002), and how the time was used leading up to the death and the care received (Finlay & Dallimore 1991, Meyer et al 2002, Seecharan et al 2004). The complexity of the bereavement process raises questions of just how wide is the range of normal bereavement? It is through the understanding of the bereavement process that pathological variants (Barrett & Scott 1989, Bowlby 1997) may be identified.

Counsellor: 'The mother believed she was coping and had moved on through much of her grief after the death of her little boy 6 years before, but when her own mother died recently after a long illness, her grief was so profound, intense and devastating that she could not function on a daily basis for a year. She came to me. It emerged that she had not accepted the death of her son, and was still in denial.'

Complicated grief can include unresolved or inhibited grief, which is delayed grief. Complicated grief is accompanied by maladaptive reactions which can be considered as pathological (Rando 1993). There is an overlap with psychiatric conditions. Some people may describe themselves as 'going mad with grief' as part of normal bereavement. However, adjustment disorders in grief include major depression, substance abuse, and states of increased anxiety with associated behaviour. There is a distinct and prolonged disruption of psychosocial functioning (Rando 1993). Bereavement is a psychological and emotional process which affects the physical and spiritual well-being of the bereaved. The bereavement process can also be experienced after traumatic loss, e.g. in paralysis, amputation, relationship breakdown. These also relate to the loss of anticipated futures, sudden and traumatic life changes, and a change in self-regard. In this way bereavement can be seen to be a process undertaken by the living of an aspect of oneself that dies.

A 10-year-old boy with a deteriorating degenerative condition commented sadly: 'I miss walking.' In deteriorating conditions there can be an ongoing loss of skills and abilities which in turn affects the sense of self of a person. If the person is a child or young person who is still developing a sense of self, this deeply affects self-esteem and positive self-image. As one 15-year-old boy said of his life: 'What's the point? I can't move. I can't do anything. I might as well finish it right now.' He presented with a flat affect and a depressive mood.

This same young man, when asked what he would like to do in life, replied that he wanted to be a professional footballer. He had been paralysed for 3 years and unable to walk for 6 years but had not changed his aspirations to accommodate his paralysis. In this way his future sense of himself and his aspirations were being lost reluctantly.

Anticipatory bereavement

Anticipatory bereavement or mourning occurs in advance of an impending loss. It occurs because the loss is anticipated and part of the grieving is already being worked through and being considered before the loss has occurred. It includes the cultural and social reactions to the expected death or loss (Knott & Wild 1986). Although there are similarities in the bereavement process, the anticipatory stages are marked by depression, a heightened concern for the dying person, a rehearsal or practice of the death with variations played out in the mind, and mental attempts at adjusting or planning how adjustments would and could be made after the loss. This is a form of bereavement in which the person or object whose loss is anticipated is still present and alive or part of the person. Anticipatory grief does not always occur because the loss is impending. It also does not denote that grief will be any easier or lessened in any way when the death or loss occurs (Corr et al 1997). There is also a sense of guilt in abandonment of the person before the loss or death occurs.

A man in his late 20s has a motorbike accident leaving him permanently paralysed in all four limbs. His wife of 4 years visits daily, hoping for some improvement and return of function and mobility of her husband. Over a period of several months this does not occur. Her husband cannot lift his arms or move his hands to hold hers. In her eyes the man she knew has died. Over the time she recognises this but cannot accept him as the same man. It is explained that when he leaves hospital he will be dependent for all of his needs. She mourns the loss of her husband who in her view has died, and begins divorce proceedings against this 'new' man she cannot live with before he leaves hospital. The wife is adamant that she cannot and will not have this man as her husband, or be responsible for his welfare in any way.

Here the loss has occurred but there has been no death. The wife anticipates that the 'death' of her active husband will occur when he returns home and is dependent upon her.

Anticipatory grief can occur in the family of a terminally ill person and inadvertently create a tension and a pressure within it. For example when a family is informed that the prognosis of a family member is x months, they prepare for this time. The person who is terminally ill may not be consciously aware of the prognosis but can become sensitive to it through the reactions of family members, which can be simultaneously both distancing and intensifying of an attachment relationship (Corr et al 1997). In this way the person with the life-limiting condition can be overwhelmed by the grief of others. In turn, this can create a withdrawal and a detachment from others leading to an isolation in dying by the ill person. There is a separating taking place, a dismantling of the attachment to others. According to different religious practices and beliefs dying alone can be perceived to be a positive experience for leaving this life and entering the next (Rinpoche 1992) or it can be viewed as tragic. The grief and anxiety of the impending death of another can fuel efforts to do something to save the life. When consent cannot be given by the affected person owing to an inability to communicate, or the child is not old enough to consent, medical interventions can be initiated. These can overrule considerations of the quality of life of the child or affected person. As Yudkin (1967) asks, 'must we rush around with tubes, injections, masks and respirators? Someone said recently that no one nowadays is allowed to die without being cured'.

The realisation of a possible loss or sense of anticipatory loss can create an anxiety, and those involved may return to an earlier emotional stage echoing the helpless infant (Guntrip 1992). This is an unconscious attempt to manage a life-threatening anxiety. This is acutely seen in children who may revert to earlier behaviours, e.g. insisting on only being fed by their mother, sucking their thumb. The transitional object of comforter toy or object is usually associated with young children but it is relevant to other, older age groups.

> Cancer patient aged 36 years: 'When I went into hospital for the start of treatment I took a couple of things which belonged to my husband and my child. I wanted the reassurance and the reminder of their presence even when they were not there. My daughter understood this completely and gave me her old teddy as she said I needed the hugs at night.'

Anticipatory bereavement can be difficult to understand when viewed at a distance by staff, as it appears neglectful and without care. It can be seen as an unconscious defensive and protective response to distance oneself from the emotional pain and trauma of seeing a loved one dying, and of the forced separation. However, this also creates a sense of abandonment for the sick person. Children are especially sensitive to this abandonment and separation in the attachment relationship. A child with no concept of time, perceives a loss of the parent when a parent does not see the child. As one healthy 5-year-old asked of her father on the telephone, 'Do you still love me Daddy?' She had not seen her father for 2 days. Judd (1995) asks if the withdrawn state of children who are dying is a defensive reaction in turn to the emotional withdrawal of the parent(s). She suggests (1995, p. 179) that this creates a 'serious emotional danger' for the children who feel alone and frightened, as if it is too frightening for the parents to face them. This is living with dying which is stressful and acutely painful.

> An 8-year-old girl with terminal cancer was given a prognosis of 2 months by the doctor. The parents were devoted to spending their time with their daughter, and rotated their working hours to be with her. When she lived into her sixth month following the prognosis the parents were becoming tired and as the mother described it, 'all strung out'. The child had deteriorated over the time and was admitted to a hospice for terminal care. The parents were adamant that they could not have their daughter back at home, and had begun to clear away her bedroom and toys. The hospice then shared care with a respite children's home until the child died some 20 weeks later at the hospice.
>
> Staff at the respite home and hospice had difficulty understanding and accepting the parents' lack of visits and apparent lack of interest in their daughter.

The prognosis can trigger a bereavement response which can be described as an anticipatory grief response creating a sense of loss. For example, a mother when given the diagnosis and prognosis for both of her daughters on the same day, said that she had lost her daughters on that day even though they were fit and active toddlers, and too that she had lost the women that they would become, and the children they would have had. The mother described life being taken away, which was the projected future loss of their lives and hers with them.

Caring for the deceased person

When someone is dying, relatives and loved ones may be present. In a hospital when the person has died the body is removed from the ward and placed in the mortuary of the hospital. When the person has died it is as if there is an abrupt end, the body is taken away, and there is no role for those left.

'My wife died in a car accident. It was a normal day in so many ways, and suddenly she wasn't there. I got to see her briefly in order to identify her, at the hospital. I never got to hold her again, nor to talk to her properly. I always felt that loss, of just being able to say goodbye properly.'

However, when a person dies at a hospice or at home there is an opportunity to care for the body, and to talk to the deceased. This is part of the bereavement process of being able to come to terms with the death. The above example is in marked contrast to the following experience at a children's hospice.

Mother of 11-year-old boy: 'My son died early in the morning at hospital. When he was close to dying the nursing staff contacted the hospice, at my request. The hospice staff all knew we were coming to the end. They asked what I would like to do. We had discussed this sometime before, and I said yes, I did want him to go over to the hospice. I didn't want to put him down. So two staff came over in an estate car. They didn't have a coffin or anything like that just blankets. I sat in the back with him in my arms and we were swaddled with these blankets to keep us warm. Although it was to keep me warm really not Tom, and to wrap Tom a little for any leakages too, but I didn't realise that at the time. We arrived at the hospice where there was a bedroom just like all the others but kept separate in another part of the building with its own entrance. There were two other staff to meet us and we went in. There were soft lights and a bed made for him with his favourite duvet cover waiting on the bed. The name-plate he had painted was on the door. I wanted to give him a bath and to change him. The staff filled a lukewarm bath and I remember checking the temperature because I didn't want it too cold. I put some oil in the bath, I bathed him, I dried and held him. I dressed him in clothes I had chosen for him. We laid him on his bed and I put some music on. His key worker was with us throughout and we had tea together. I didn't want to be apart from him. I sat on the sofa in the room looking out onto the little garden. My other son, who was 17 then, came along too, and we sat and hugged. He hugged his little brother and gave him a kiss goodnight. I stayed in a bedroom up the stair and could go down and check on Tom all the time. There was always a little light on all through the night for him. Tom and I stayed at the hospice for 5 days. Since my husband had died I was on my own. The staff helped me to arrange the funeral, and also helped me to contact relatives and friends to tell them Tom had died. They made the tea when visitors came when we sat in the separate sitting room. Over those days

Tom became cold and stiff. It was so difficult, but I came to realise he was dead. At the beginning I always wanted to hold him, but over those days it was enough to stroke his cheek, and touch his hand. But he was so very cold, and he looked different. I could see Tom had gone.

'His gran was upset to see him but she said it had helped her as she had last seen him when he was alive, and would not have believed he had died. His granddad didn't want to see him but said he would remember him alive.

'On the day Tom was put into his coffin and the lid put on, I said my last goodbye. Before we left the hospice for the funeral that day the staff held a little service to say goodbye to Tom. All the people who knew him came to say goodbye including the secretary and the cook. I went back to the hospice after 2 weeks and sat in that special room and thought of Tom. I sat with Janet, his key worker, and we shared memories of times with Tom. She had some photos for me of Tom at the hospice too. That was lovely. I go back to the hospice now on the anniversary of his death and say a little hallo and goodbye to him. When I think of the day he died, I know I did everything for him on that day. It was a good day in so many ways, but so painful. I was helped through it, and I could say goodbye in my way.'

At the children's hospice it was recognised that the care and love do not end, but if thwarted contribute to further distress. Not everyone feels able to carry out all the tasks this mother felt compelled to do for her child, nor is it appropriate, but she was supported in what she wanted to do. Everyone is different. In palliative care it is understood that there is a life-limiting condition, and this can provide an opportunity to sensitively discuss what people would like to have happen when they die. The person often already has wishes but has felt unable to discuss them with anyone, for fear of being perceived as morbid. This can be true of family too, 'as if by talking about it I might be tempting providence,' confided one wife.

Palliative care is for the person and family and extends beyond life to encompass the death and bereavement. The role of the hospice can provide support at this special time of dying and death, to the loved ones of the deceased, but it is helpful to have a plan, even though this might change at the time. Cultural and religious beliefs and practices need to be ascertained before the death. For example, for a Moslem family the burial must take place within 24 hours of the death, so a plan needs to be known to avoid unnecessary stress and panic for the family. For a Buddhist there is a practice to be carried out, ideally at the time of death. For some families the body of the deceased is moved near to their home to a funeral parlour, or on the evening before the funeral the coffin and body are moved to the home. This time at, and just after, death can help those bereaved to find a meaning and purpose in the person's life, with dignity and respect, and an opportunity to show care and love in the final goodbye. This can help the bereaved in a positive way. The way in which someone can be helped at the time of death, and just afterwards, is personal and there is no defined 'right' way.

For many there is a financial difficulty in bereavement, and help needed in the financial affairs of the deceased, which needs guidance. These can be discussed with the social worker for advice regarding benefits for the bereaved, which are available.

Bereavement support

Many hospices extend bereavement support through the social worker or chaplain visiting the bereaved at home. The key worker is often involved too in the early stages (1–6 months) through visits or phone calls. As discussed, everyone is different in bereavement, some preferring to work through it themselves, others to link with a bereavement counsellor from a hospice or a voluntary organisation such as CRUSE, or a counsellor. Some of the children's hospices provide bereavement support for the whole family with parallel support groups for siblings and parents. The Seasons for Growth programme is a helpful guided course planned for adults, and children of different ages, who have experienced the death of someone. For some families a memorial or charitable event in the person's name can provide a meaning and purpose for the family in their bereavement of the loved one.

As bereavement is understood not to be a fixed-term process there is no definite cut-off time when bereavement and mourning end. It is up to individuals to determine when they no longer need support. Comments such as, 'Isn't it time you got over this?' and 'I think you are making too much of this now' tend to be a reflection of the speaker not the bereaved, and are not helpful.

At the start of life there is a positive welcome, and at death there needs to be time to say goodbye well. Both are significant events and mark our beginning and ending. Death is a normal process of life and a certainty, for nothing is permanent, although there is often denial and avoidance of talking about it even when it is close. This reluctance to discuss death can isolate the dying and the bereaved, which seems so unkind and unnecessary.

> *If we can live with the knowledge that death is our constant companion, traveling on our left shoulder, then death can become . . . our ally, still fearsome but continually a source of wise counsel . . . When we shy away from death, the ever-changing nature of things, we inevitably shy away from life.*

(Scott Peck 1990)

References

Bailley S E, Kral M J, Dunham K 1999 Survivors of suicide do grieve differently: empirical support for a common sense proposition. Suicide & Life-threatening Behavior 29(3):256–271

Barrett T W, Scott T B 1989 Development of the Grief Experience Questionnaire. Suicide & Life-threatening Behavior 19(2):201–215

Bowlby J 1997 Attachment and loss. Volume 3. Loss: sadness depression. Pimlico, London

Corr C A, Nabe C M, Corr D M 1997 Death and dying, life and living. 2nd edn. Pacific Brooks Cole, New York

Finlay I, Dallimore D 1991 Your child is dead. British Medical Journal 302(6791): 1524–15355

Freud S 1991 Mourning and melancholia. In: On metapsychology. Penguin Books, London, vol 11, p 252

Greenstreet W 2004 Why nurses need to understand the principles of bereavement theory. British Journal of Nursing 13(10):590

Guntrip H 1992 The manic–depressive problem in the light of the schizoid process. Schizoid phenomena, object relations and the self. Karnac, London

Harwood D, Hawton K, Hope T et al 2002 The grief experiences and needs of bereaved relatives and friends of older people dying through suicide: a descriptive and case-control study. Journal of Affective Disorders 72(2):185–194

Judd D 1995 Give sorrow words. Whurr, London

Knott J E, Wild E 1986 Anticipatory grief and reinvestment. In: Rando T A (ed) Loss and grief. Lexington Books, USA, pp 55–60

Martin T, Doka K 2000 Men don't cry . . . women do: transcending gender stereotypes of grief. Psychology Press (UK), London

Meyer E C, Burns J P, Griffith J L et al 2002 Parental perspectives on end of life care in the pediatric intensive care unit. Critical Care Medicine 30(1): 226–231

Parkes C M 1972 Bereavement: studies of grief in adult life. International Universities Press, New York

Rando T A 1993 Treatment of complicated mourning. Research Press, Champaign

Rinpoche S 1992 The Tibetan book of living and dying. Rider, London

Scott Peck M 1990 The road less travelled. Arrow, London, pp 142–143

Seecharan G A, Andresen E M, Norris K et al 2004 Parents' assessment of quality of care and grief following a child's death. Archives of Pediatrics & Adolescent Medicine 158(6):515–520

Stroebe M, Schut H 1999 The dual process model of coping with bereavement: rationale and description. Death Studies 23(3):197

Thesaurus 2006 Online. Available: http://www. Thesaurus.reference.com

Walter T 1996 A new model of grief; bereavement and biography. Mortality 1(1):7–25

Yudkin S 1967 Children and death. Lancet 1:37–41

Suggested further reading

Christ G H, Christ A E 2006 Current approaches to helping children cope with a parent's terminal illness. A Cancer Journal for Clinicians 56:197–212. Online. Available: http://www.caonline. amcancersoc.org 2 Sept 2006

Central DuPage Hospital 2006 Care of the terminally ill child. Series. Online. Available: http://www. cdh.org/HealthInformation 31 Oct 2006

Harrison S, Weiss L 1996 My book about me. Greenfield Publishing, Kenilworth. Available from The Child Bereavement Trust (see under Organisations below)

Jacob S 1996 The grief experience of older women whose husbands had hospice care. Journal of Advanced Nursing 24:280–286

The Bereavement Risk Assessment, an assessment tool used by some hospices to identify areas of need and behaviour for the bereaved, is based upon this work

Levy L H 1992 Anticipatory grief its measurement and proposed reconceptualization. The Hospice Journal 7(4):1–28

Mazanec P, Tyler M K 2003 Cultural considerations in end-of-life care. American Journal of Nursing 103(3):50–58

Not My Kid website 2006 Common reactions to grief/loss. Online. Available: http://www.notmykid. org/parentArticles/Grief/default.asp 2 Sep 2006

People Living with Cancer website 2005 Helping a child or teenager who is grieving. Online. Available: http://www.plwc.org 2 Sept 2006

Rando T A (ed) 1985 Parental loss of a child. Research Press, Champaign

Rando T A 1991 How to go on living when someone you love dies. Updated paperback version of Grieving: how to go on living when someone you love dies. Bantam Press, New York

Rando T A 2006 Therapeutic interventions in grief and mourning – home study programme. Online. Available: http://www.jkseminars.com/randoce.html 31 Oct 2006

Some organisations

BACP (British Association for Counselling and Psychotherapy). Information available from: http://www.bacp.co.uk

Child Bereavement Network. National resource for bereaved children and young people. Information available from; http://www.ncb.org.uk/cbn

The Child Bereavement Trust. Provides training, information and support for professionals working with bereaved parents and children. The telephone helpline number is: 0845 357 1000. Information available from: http://www.childbereavement.org.uk

Citizens Advice. Available from ; http://www. citizenadvice.org.uk

Macmillan Cancer Relief. Information on resources and publications including professional resources. Available at: http://www.Macmillan.org.uk

Marie Curie Cancer Care. Information on leaflets available, advice and publications. Information available from: http://www.mariecurie.org.uk

RIPRAP. An interactive website for teenagers who have a parent with cancer. http://www.riprap.org.uk

Seasons for Growth programme originates from Australia where it is also known as Good Grief. Information available from http://www.goodgrief.org.au/nav.htm

Information on adult and children's programmes available from UK distribution centre for materials and training at Notre Dame Centre, Scotland, email: sfg@notredamecentre.org.uk

Winstons Wish. Provides a family helpline, information and support for parents and carers of bereaved children. Available from: http://www.winstonswish.org.uk

Appendix 6.1
Bereavement support for children

6.1

Claire Tester

Children's hospices provide bereavement support to families including children. Some support may be through a group for children which runs alongside the parent group. These are still new. Having worked for 7 years in a bereavement group for children I have found some central tenets to be helpful in holding a successful group for children. These are broadly:

- Same leaders for the group for familiarity and trust.
- A contained regular setting, not a thoroughfare area.
- Same time, same length of time, and a defined end – with a clock to help.
- No disturbances or interruptions from staff or other children.
- Understood group rules are set, and reminded each time in regard to respect and listening.
- Acceptance of some children remaining quiet.
- Siblings are kept together in the same group.
- Very small children and infants have a supported separate session, which is through play.
- Parallel group with parents beginning all together for welcome then general introduction to session, going into separate groups in different room, then joining together at defined time for cakes and drinks – comfort food.
- An identified beginning, middle and end to any group.
- A planned activity with something made/drawn etc.
- Child-friendly objects such as choice of crayons, paints, pens, coloured paper, etc. and comfortable informal seating, e.g. big cushions.
- Nice snacks and drinks available and shared.
- Adolescents may start at the beginning but need to be taken to a separate room for the 'middle' of the session, apart from younger children, rejoining at the end.
- Activities also focus on the importance of the living children, so that they are not defined as 'bereaved siblings'.
- Activities and opportunities for expression and sharing.
- Importance of being active, which can include a planned bolt for the door and a game outside, e.g. hide and seek is popular – can you see me? can you find me in all this grief?
- No coaxing or goading children to speak.
- Something tangible is made to take home.
- Understanding by parents of the child's needs, not just seen as playing.
- Importance of using festival times in the year. As one mother said, 'Thank you for the Easter egg hunt, I just can't deal with it this year and she loves it.'
- Acceptance that children may not be consistent attenders because parents cannot come, or the child does not want to go that week.

- Regular sessions, but only every 10–12 weeks or so, which links with ends of term times.
- To maintain a link with children or young people by giving a contact number that they can use, or may choose not to use. They are not telephoned, you are.
- Shared feedback with children to parents at end with staff support.
- Planning and feedback time for staff to discuss.

It depends upon the nature of the group, whether it is for a specified number of sessions, or if it is a long-term ongoing group, as to how activities are planned. For example, the Seasons for Growth programme has a set course with books to accompany the course.

Bereavement groups for children involve play, but are not about playing. There is a balance between an activity about thinking and sharing what has happened to them, trying to understand the process and putting questions in a supported environment; and having opportunities to reaffirm their own identity, individuality and strengths as well as hopes and dreams for their future.

Section 2

Creative interventions

Counselling skills – painting a clearer picture

Kathryn Boog

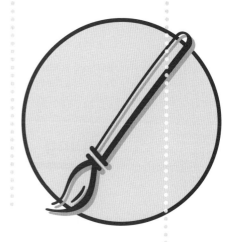

Life is like a tin of sardines – we are all looking for the key.

Alan Bennett

Key words

changed agenda; challenges; relationships; therapeutic relationship; Pandora's box; life review

7

Supporting people to establish a good quality of living in their final few weeks and days begins with the quest to discover what matters most and what they want to achieve in that time. This is often a combination of practical and emotional matters, which intertwine with, and influence each other, and good palliative care will involve helping patients as they sift and sort through this melting pot of symptoms, feelings and constantly changing circumstances.

As the disease process enters its final stage, and function declines, the focus of attention changes from the physical issues relating to comfort and control, to those of a psychological, emotional and spiritual nature. Concerns over how to manage activities of daily living, despite the limitations imposed by a variety of symptoms, are gradually replaced by existential issues. An increasing awareness of impending death stimulates the need to evaluate life's roles and achievements, and to consolidate an existence. Goals and activities related to dying take precedence – how to say goodbye, making arrangements for others to be able to cope on a practical level or making funeral plans, for example. People may feel that they are no longer the person they once were, and are struggling to recognise something of their old selves, with their hopes and dreams, in this person with terminal disease. They may ask themselves: who am I; where have I come from; what have I done with my life; how will I be remembered? The realisation that there is little time left to influence these issues throws everything into sharp perspective and may cause anxiety and distress, whilst the re-evaluation of what is important in life, refocusing on new priorities and reframing the approach towards achieving these new goals, can be a complex and overwhelming task.

Coping

A number of factors such as personality, previous experiences or the nature of a relationship can affect the ability of individuals to cope with their circumstances and their experience of dying, and whilst some people may be aware of these influences, others can feel overwhelmed by their situation and unable to see the reasons for their distress. The result can be a style of coping that is difficult for others to deal with, where individuals become withdrawn, uncommunicative, demanding, clingy or obsessive (Lugton 2002), putting pressure on one carer or wanting only one member of staff to work with them.

Jean had always seemed very nervous and insecure. When she was feeling ill, she became child-like, wanting everything done for her and needing to be coaxed to participate in any activities or even to eat and drink. During the relaxation sessions, she needed something to cuddle – a cushion or a soft toy – and it was noted that when she was completely absorbed in this activity, she relaxed, and a smile was always there. At the end of each session, Jean was keen to share her imagery with the others in the group – it was always related to a holiday that she had had at the seaside, with her mother, when she was about 8 years old. She was reluctant, though, to reveal anything much more about her childhood despite encouragement from the therapist and the others in the group. However, just after she arrived one morning she burst into tears and, with the therapist guiding the conversation, began to talk about an incident from her childhood. Her mother had been killed in a fatal accident and Jean felt she had been responsible for the death because of a casual remark that she had made that day to a friend. She had carried this burden with her throughout her life and now that she was dying herself, it was troubling her even more. She wanted to be the child she was before that terrible day, to return to a time when she felt safe and happy. Jean was encouraged to talk to the clinical psychologist about her feelings, and after several sessions she was much more settled and felt able to cope with her present circumstances.

Another coping style that can be challenging is when the patient adopts the sick role. If the reasons for this situation can be revealed and understood, such as the secondary benefits to the patient of this type of behaviour, then the reasons for non-compliance with a treatment programme will become apparent and can be addressed.

Patients may experience anxiety, guilt or fear as a symptom – such as pain or breathlessness – and if they do not relate their feelings to their physical discomfort, control of those particular symptoms can be difficult (Lichter 1991).

Examination of individual priorities will reveal their unique significance to the patient, and they are usually a combination of practical and emotional issues. Practical concerns will include maintaining independence in activities of daily living; continuing with social and family activities – which will be influenced by cultural and ethnic factors – and using this time to 'get things in order', such as tying up financial and legal dealings, for example, or planning the funeral. Saying goodbye and leaving gifts, cards and letters are examples of goals influenced by emotional needs, as is the desire for reconciliation and the need for people to know that they will not be forgotten.

This is reflected in the increasing importance of relationship issues that can have a major influence on patients' day-to-day well-being and the complexity of their symptoms.

Some people feel that they want to keep going for as long as possible in their familiar roles, because to let go, or change, can be perceived as a threat to personhood and a loss of control. This, added to the other losses already incurred – of physical or mental ability, body image, of the role within their social group and of their future – will present a challenging situation, causing anger and resentment, which can become demoralising and hopeless, resulting in a poor quality of life.

By assisting in the process of reviewing, refining and redirecting the individual's goals, professionals can empower patients to meet these challenges, regain some control in areas of their lives that are important to them, and offer the opportunity for personal growth.

Understanding attitudes

Using counselling skills whilst individuals are telling their life story will enhance the understanding of patients' complex and subjective perspectives of themselves and their situation. Listening to feelings and reflecting them back allows both patient and professional to view the meaning of the illness experience in the context of the patient's life story. The real person behind the illness – that person's strengths and weaknesses, individual philosophy, roles and personal drivers – can be revealed, and achievements acknowledged, increasing feelings of self-worth and improving self-esteem. Personal stories may also give some indication of attitudes and coping strategies and the relationship between past issues and present behaviour, perhaps explaining the reason for failure to comply with a treatment programme. They can also provide the opportunity for feelings of doubt, shame, guilt or regret to be expressed.

Amelia had given all her energies to her career, to provide what she considered was the best possible upbringing for her only child. Jenny had wanted for nothing as far as her mother could see, but as death approached, Amelia felt lonely and sad. Jenny's visits were few and far between and when she did come, the atmosphere was tense, filling Amelia with despair. It became apparent to Amelia that her daughter had felt abandoned and hurt as a child. Her mother had rarely been around at times when Jenny felt she should have been there, and now she was to be left alone again. Amelia still had all the drawings and letters that her daughter had sent her over the years when she was travelling, and told the therapist how much she had treasured these. She did not regret her past and wanted Jenny to understand her reasons for her lifestyle. Together, Amelia and the therapist created a story album of her life and included the things that her daughter had sent. Amelia presented this to her daughter and through the sharing of experiences they began to understand more about each other and to accept the situation for the way it was. Together, and with the help of the therapist, they worked on the content of the order of service for Amelia's funeral that concluded with the playing of the Edith Piaf song, 'No Regrets'.

All of this information can be used to ensure a meaningful and purposeful experience for the patient who is terminally ill, but the value of that information, its interpretation and the patient's subsequent compliance in the treatment programme, will be influenced by the quality of the therapeutic relationship. Good interaction will result when facilitators are comfortable with the technique, have insight into their own life's narrative, and can use their own life skills and experience to enhance their personal coping strategy. In this way, the therapeutic use of self, involving self-awareness and the use of appropriate self-disclosure, will encourage patients to reveal their innermost thoughts and feelings.

However, professionals' attitude to illness, dying and death, and fears of confronting these issues, can result in feelings of anxiety and insecurity. They may feel compromised and vulnerable, resulting in a superficial interaction where cues are deliberately misread, or diversionary tactics are used to avoid the issues arising (Burton 1991).

Encouraging patients to participate in activity sessions in order to distract them from distressing or difficult thoughts, is one such tactic sometimes used as a defence mechanism (Job et al 1997). Other common distancing techniques include switching to another subject or delegating responsibility to someone else; keeping the topic of conversation on neutral ground; offering encouragement or reassurance at the wrong time, and for the wrong reasons; and trying to offer solutions to problems before hearing the full story.

A further barrier to good communication is presuming that the patient will mention something with little or no prompting if it is really important, as is making the assumption that it would take too long either to find out the information, or to deal with any issues disclosed. There may also be a feeling that there would be no support available, either for the patient or the professional, should complex and painful issues arise, and so – do we open Pandora's box, and if we do, can we deal with the consequences? This question is relevant to both the patient and the professional, and either can have control over the answer.

Using a counselling technique

Points to consider

- The aim is to develop a holistic view of individuals, and to help them to sift through and sort out issues affecting their well-being.
- The approach should be humanistic and person-centred.
- Giving quality time and not rushing the interaction will encourage a relaxed mood.
- Facilitators need to adopt a comfortable and open position, giving the patient their full attention.
- Be consistent in the messages that are given to the patient – body language and dialogue must have congruence. This will help in the development of the therapeutic relationship (Burton 1991).
- Instil confidence, trust, control, and assure the patient of confidentiality.
- Be prepared to listen more than talk. Skilful listening in a relaxed and supportive environment will make it easier for people to express themselves and their problems.
- Use a sensitive and non-judgmental approach.
- Identify people's strengths and underline the positives in their stories.
- Allow comfortable silences.
- Use touch, eye contact and appropriate humour as communication aids.

The intervention/technique for promoting disclosure

- Start with an open, directive question: 'What did you feel when he said . . . ?'
- Follow with a mixture of open and closed questions.
- Review what you feel the person has said and reflect that back: 'So you were feeling . . . because . . . ?' Using a tentative response will allow the patient to either agree with, or correct you.

- Clarify: 'Could you tell me what you mean by . . . ?'
- Encourage precision: 'When exactly did you notice that feeling?'
- Empathise with the person. Consider how you might feel in that situation: 'That sounds terrible for you.' 'I can see that that would make you angry.'
- Follow and lead as necessary.
- Allow silences, followed by: 'We can come back to that later.'
- Summarise and screen periodically.
- If unsure of the meaning of something that has been said, repeat the last few words, in question format: 'So you're not quite sure what they meant?'
- If the person cries, say: 'It's all right to cry. Sometimes that's what you need to do – to just let go of these feelings.'
- Bring the interview to a close: 'We will need to finish very shortly, is there anything else you would like to tell me, that you feel you've missed out?'
- Thank the patient for sharing something personal with you.

Attention to cues

- Careful observation of patients' body language and observation of their behaviour during the conversation will help distinguish what is really being said. 'People's silent comments often speak volumes' (Hume 1999).
- Be sensitive to picking up distress signals.
- Be aware of unconscious communication and contradictory messages.

Non-verbal cues may include:

- posture – slouching, head hung low
- fidgeting/restlessness/agitation
- poor eye contact, or lack of it
- wringing hands
- pulling at clothes
- excessive swallowing
- rapid breathing or breathlessness.

Verbal cues may involve:

- testing – to see if everyone's stories are the same
- throw-away lines: 'They say I only have a few weeks,' or 'I'm thinking of going to Australia to see my son next Christmas.'

Counselling skills can be used in a variety of ways

- Deliberate manipulation of the conversation, where the professional is directing and influencing the content.
- Seizing the opportunity to develop the situation – in response to other cues such as body language, eye contact/lack of eye contact.
- During other interventions such as assessment, activities of daily living practice, creativity sessions and using the activity as a catalyst to encourage disclosure.
- Following an activity session – relaxation, reminiscence.
- Alongside psychodynamic activity such as relaxation, where the dialogue used can encourage catharsis (Liossi & Mystakidou 1997).

- During reminiscence sessions and life review where the emotional release offered by disclosure and the sharing of concerns can be a liberating experience.

Life review

Life-story work, reminiscence and life review all share the traits of acknowledgement of personhood, affirmation of positive past actions and experiences, and the opportunity to share that person's unique contribution to life – who the person is, where the person came from, and how the person got there. They acknowledge personal achievements, good feelings and improved self-worth and a sense of belonging, acknowledging the person's place in time, role and self-identity, offering hope for the future, based on the positives uncovered. Personal stories can be developed into life-story books and memory albums, ensuring that patients will be remembered in the way that they would want – another positive outcome from this activity.

Reminiscence and life-story work may also uncover negative issues from the past, but whilst these are offered as regrets, they may not directly affect people's ability to accept the past and move on with their life. Where resolution has not occurred, and the patient is unable to relegate these experiences to the past and move on, life review should be considered as a therapeutic intervention. It is an individual process, a focused activity in which the therapist, through structured questioning and the use of counselling skills, encourages the patient to revisit specific times in the past. In this situation, unresolved issues can be identified and retrospectively evaluated, empowering patients to accept their past actions as the only way it could have been.

Colin, who had lost touch with his son and wanted to explain his circumstances and past actions and reinstate his relationship with his son: 'I thought doing the life story was a bit of a farce until I told my son about it – he wanted a copy and was thrilled when he saw it. He left for Canada when he was 21 and I think that doing the life story . . . has been the means that brought us together again.'

Aspects for young people and children

These are discussed in Chapter 9, and in Appendix 6.1 on bereavement support for children and Appendix 12.4 on therapeutic communication with children.

References

Burton M 1991 In: Watson M (ed) Cancer patient care: psychosocial treatment methods. BPS Books, Cambridge, pp 75–85

Hume C 1999 Spirituality: a part of total care? British Journal of Occupational Therapy 62(8):367–370

Job T, Broom W, Habermehl F 1997 Coming out! Time to acknowledge the importance of counselling skills in occupational therapy. British Journal of Occupational Therapy 60(8):357–358

Lichter I 1991 Some psychological causes of distress in the terminally ill. Palliative Medicine 5:138–146

Liossi C, Mystakidou K 1997 Catharsis in palliative care. European Journal of Palliative Care 4(4):133–136

Lugton J 2002 Communicating with dying people and their relatives. Radcliffe Medical Press, Oxford

Creativity

Kathryn Boog

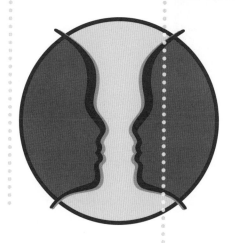

Creativity is the ability to use skills to bring into existence something that wasn't there before or change something that is ... It involves having the confidence to work with a number of known or unknown variables to manifest a solution.

The Scotsman **1 March 2006**

Key words

control; identity; rehabilitation; leisure; communication; expression; legacy; symptom control; lateral thinking

8

In the face of terminal illness, the re-establishment of previous occupations can help patients to regain control over their lives (Vrkljan & Miller-Polgar 2001). Functional disabilities are acknowledged and accommodated by the therapist in the pursuit of the patient's need to maintain a satisfying and stimulating existence, but with increasingly debilitating symptoms rehabilitation in the normally accepted sense of the word becomes less of an option, and creative and lateral thinking will be required in order to maintain occupational roles and identity. Patients retain their autonomy when they are still able to make choices – which activities to participate in, when and how. Even when the patient is very limited by disease the possibility still exists for a sense of achievement and control to be established. Activities can be adapted in order to make them still possible, and to allow continued participation, although in a different way.

Being creative can allow the individual to continue to do things that are meaningful by adapting established activities and developing replacements to still engender the same feelings and fulfil the same needs as those that are no longer achievable. Physical limitations can be sidestepped when the therapist becomes the patient's 'hands' (Nainis et al 2005), carrying out the process by following their directions and therefore allowing them to retain control.

Creativity may be viewed as a complement to other, more well-established forms of rehabilitation, using the arts to discover hidden, or unacknowledged talents in order to maintain a person's sense of self, and to achieve precious goals and reinstate feelings of having some control no matter how compromised the person's abilities might be.

Ann talking about silk painting: 'In the beginning I didn't feel that I could do anything by myself. But with the scarf, it began to be that I was in control.'

Reviewing their occupational history with patients, will provide the therapist with an insight into which activities have been significant to the individual, and why. How these assumed roles are linked to the formation and continuity of the individual's identity, including cultural and existential influences, will direct the choice of appropriate alternative activities, restoring a sense of control through these, and helping to restore feelings of accomplishment, and of moving on, promoting a more positive outlook. Changing the emphasis from the things that the person is unable to do, to focusing on what is still possible, will be a fulfilling experience, guiding that person towards a sense of satisfaction in achievement.

Choosing to pursue a creative activity that the patient has done very well prior to illness is not always a good idea. Whilst it is possible to use positioning, and modify activities, this can underline patients' inability to perform the task to their previous standards and satisfaction, the end result seeming inferior and unacceptable to them. Past artwork can be developed and new items produced from it, perpetuating the feelings of accomplishment associated with the originals.

Carrie had always been a poor sleeper. She taught herself to paint as a way to while away the hours during the night and used painting as a way to help relax her in times of stress. Fatigue was making this difficult now and she was unhappy with her attempts to paint, but she still needed to feel creative. She brought her favourite paintings into the day hospice and they were scanned into the computer and used to make cards that she wanted to be sold in the hospice shop.

People still need to feel useful, and that they can still learn new things. The stimulation of a new challenge and the concentration required in order to master it will provide relief from the constant negative thoughts surrounding the illness. Participation allows for enjoyment of the moment and surprise at the realisation of how quickly time has passed (Reynolds & Prior 2006), and a successful outcome will engender feelings of control (Nainis et al 2005), replacing lost abilities and fostering a positive mood. The surprise discovery of a creative talent provides a positive element amidst a sea of negative experiences, fostering a sense of achievement and accomplishment.

Ken, day hospice: 'Before you try you're afraid of it. You make excuses like my hand's not steady; I'm no good at colours. You're afraid to make a mess, but once you begin you're really motoring and you never go back because you're always improving yourself.'

Creativity can be enjoyed for its own merits, unfettered by the need to conform, or to perform at a certain level or in a particular way (Obrian 2001, Thompson & Blair 1998). It encourages self-expression, underlining and maintaining individuality and reflecting cultural and spiritual identity. The person behind the illness, and the unique qualities that make that person, can be shown, helping with regaining and maintaining a sense of who that person is (Howie et al 2004) and reinstating self-esteem and restoring dignity.

The side effects of treatments made Fiona feel bloated. She had lost her beautiful auburn hair, and cerebral involvement meant that her communication skills were poor. She desperately wanted staff to know her as the person she was – a successful playwright and friend of the rich and famous. Together with the therapist, Fiona made a collage that included photos and newspaper cuttings of reviews of her plays, and articles about her from well-known magazines. The collage was hung in her room, stimulating a lot of memories and conversation as people recognised her, much to her delight.

Artwork can be used to personalise space, either around the bed in an inpatient unit, or in the person's rooms at home (Bye 1998).

Wilma had spent a lot of time in her new conservatory. She wanted to surround herself with images of her favourite things and so she made a collage of summer flowers from her garden and painted glass roundels with bright colours to remind her of the warm days of summer.

Existential issues/influences

Creativity can be used by people to confirm their existence (Perrin 2001) now and in the future, by aiding generativity and legacy, transcending death by leaving something of themselves behind (Chochinov et al 2005). The created object may be left as a legacy, thereby assuring continuity of that person's existence into the future and for generations to come. The legacies left behind can help in the grieving process as people adjust to their loss (Obrian 2001).

It can be used to confirm relationships and to establish, in a tangible way, emotions which had been assumed to be understood, or may never have been voiced. Created objects can aid communication where talking is difficult, and provide an opportunity to make amends or to acknowledge acceptance of a past situation. They are symbols, representing the creator's innermost thoughts and feelings.

In the face of deteriorating health, people begin to review and evaluate their life, as its psychological and existential aspects become ever more important (Allied Health Professions Palliative Care Project Team 2004). The complex relationships and interactions between the different aspects of an individual's life are pushed to the fore, influencing the dying experience. Creative expression, as a psychodynamic activity, can be a powerful means of addressing these (Boog 2006). It enables the externalisation of feelings where it is difficult to use the spoken word – either because it would be too painful or uncomfortable, or because of cognitive difficulties or communication issues, such as aphasia (Devlin 2006).

There may be expressions of regret or guilt at the outcome of past actions and people may feel that they would like to make amends, or to regenerate relationships that have been lost. A creative approach can help them to make these connections, providing complementary symptom relief, making the problem more manageable, and allowing patients the chance to control and influence these aspects of their existence and consolidate their lives. Where verbal interaction is difficult, feelings can be expressed non-verbally, by using the written word or by creating an object as a symbolic representation of those sentiments.

> Paul was desolate. The previous evening he had lost his temper at his son and told him never to come back. The therapist talked through the events and helped Paul to see that it was his illness and his situation that he was angry with. He would never see his son grow into a man, feel proud when he graduated from university, or hold his grandchild. Despite his exhaustion, Paul was able to make a card for his son, using a simple collage to decorate the front and, with help, chose some words to explain his outburst.

The desire to be remembered in a positive way is equally important where relationships have been good. People want to ensure that significant information is recorded for posterity and that those dearest to them are aware of their feelings. They may want to be remembered at a significant future event where they would ordinarily have played a role, such as a wedding or a child's birthday, or to feel that tradition is continued at family occasions.

> Norma knew she would not see her daughter married, but wanted to make sure that she could take part in the preparations. She made the favours for the dining tables and designed the invitations on the computer, with the help of the therapist.

This may again involve the written word or the making of gifts that will be left as a legacy. The objects will all have symbolic meaning, and will represent the feelings and the care that went into their creation.

Symptom management

Control of symptoms may be difficult to achieve because of influences other than the disease or its treatments. The most common symptoms – fatigue, breathlessness, pain and nausea – can be exacerbated by anxieties related to a variety of influences, e.g. emotional, spiritual, social and relationship issues.

Patients report a decrease in a variety of symptoms following creative activity sessions, notably fatigue, which may be related to feelings of relief at being distracted for a while from their negative thoughts about their illness (Nainis et al 2005). Being engrossed in an activity can help with other symptoms, such as pain, breathlessness and nausea, where there is an element of anxiety preventing an acceptable level of relief. In this way, the deep concentration involved in being totally absorbed in the activity, acts as a non-pharmacological method of symptom management, referred to as 'flow' in the literature (Wright 2004).

The relationship between levels of discomfort and weakness, and the ability to participate in activity, can be completely disproportionate when the patient is 'driven' to complete a task that has great personal meaning. Fatigue levels appear to diminish (Nainis et al 2005) so that, when they wish to complete unfinished business and effect emotional closure, even the most exhausted patients can somehow muster the energy to engage, albeit for short spells, in order to complete their objective.

This change in the reported experience of fatigue may in part be due to engagement in a purposeful activity where the patient had felt this was no longer possible, relieving the lethargy and boredom experienced by some at the end of life.

Boredom is a symptom often overlooked in the care of the terminally ill. People become frustrated and demoralised as their attempts to continue their previous lifestyles are systematically thwarted. Lack of energy, breathlessness and pain make it difficult, if not impossible to deal with important and significant issues, causing anxiety and despondency. Multiple and continuing losses can lead to a lack of purpose and a sense of loneliness (Brown & McKenna 1999) and despair.

People who have previously led active lives, and who have had little time for leisure pursuits, may now find time heavy on their hands and need to find something to do to fill the void that is left. Enforced occupational deprivation, due to lack of energy both to physically manage previous activities and be able to concentrate for any length of time, may be another reason for the boredom, frustration and demoralisation often experienced by this patient group. A different kind of rehabilitation, using creative solutions (Peloquin 1997) will be a useful means of addressing these negative feelings, the act of creativity itself becoming the tool of choice.

The challenge of learning the new task and mastering it will encourage the patient to develop other new skills, providing stimulation and counteracting boredom (Reynolds & Prior 2006) and the weariness (Cassidy 1991) and lethargy often mistaken for boredom. Taking steps to ensure that the experience – that is, both the activity and the outcome – is a positive one, will encourage further participation, helping to provide respite from this common but rarely acknowledged symptom.

Molly: 'If you're feeling down and you're in that mood that you can't be bothered, you concentrate so much on what you're doing that you forget that you're down in the mouth.'

Creativity as a therapeutic tool

Creative activity can be used as a catalyst in the therapeutic situation where working together with the therapist on a project will provide patients with the opportunity to express themselves and their feelings, both verbally and non-verbally (Fisher et al 1997, Thompson & Blair 1998). Skilful listening, using counselling skills, and encouraging trust, will help patients to feel at ease and comfortable and thus able to express themselves and their concerns more easily. The professional can be directive or follow the patients' lead, as appropriate.

Working alongside patients in artwork will provide the opportunity for them to express feelings, air emotions and problems, and identify strengths and positives, whilst listening to, and reading, the prose and poetry of others will enhance the therapeutic relationship. Having empathy with the patient allows the professional to acknowledge the patient's situation, and to suggest appropriate creative activities to address important issues. This is particularly relevant when helping with last gifts, poetry, card making, writing transcripts of life stories and in producing an order of service for the funeral. It allows the professional to direct (Rahman 2000) patients towards their goal and the selection of words that are apt for their circumstances.

Constantly reviewing the process involved in carrying out the activity, and relating it to the person's deteriorating ability, will allow the professional to make adjustments and accommodate the changes, ensuring that the outcome of the activity remains the same. Difficulties performing creative activities will indicate that there are problems with functional activities such as activities of daily living (Holland 1984) where concentration, eyesight, fatigue, pain, sequencing, planning, pacing, prioritising, etc. may be compromised.

Creative activities can form part of a lifestyle management programme, introducing planning, pacing and prioritising as a concept that can then be extended into personal and domestic activities.

Approach

- Encourage empathy and trust. People will only share their precious hopes and goals with someone in whom they feel they can have confidence.
- Listen to their stories. These will give valuable clues about people and their relationships, their needs and their dreams.
- Offer guidance – how they might be able to express themselves, how to find the right words. Offer a variety of ways in which their aims can be achieved; be prepared to change direction as the situation dictates.
- Capture the moment. Be aware of deterioration in their condition, both mentally and physically, changing the length or frequency of sessions as necessary. This might mean seeing them for several very short periods throughout the day, or for one or two longer sessions when they are more aware and able to interact.
- Be flexible and prepared to drop everything to see particular patients, even for a very short time, when they feel able to engage.
- Liaise with other members of the multidisciplinary team for the best time to see the patient, and ask them to call.
- Ask patients when they feel is the best time of day for you to see them – to fit in with other activities, visitors, energy levels.
- Ensure that privacy, if required, is available and adhered to. People need to be given space, with staff being informed that they do not want to share this experience. Writers should be reassured that if their work is transcribed, it will only be viewed by themselves and the person doing the transcription, and that any preparatory documentation will be destroyed once the finished article is produced. Folders should be provided to store the work, and care should be taken when approaching the patient in the inpatient unit if there are visitors around, so that nothing is said that will give a hint about the activity.
- Artwork should be stored in individual trays.
- Participation in group work, and observing others, will instil confidence. The dynamics of a group can help people feel supported as they try new activities (Devlin 2006), and seeing the finished projects displayed will encourage people to want to participate.

Method

- Use simple, recognisable materials to instil confidence.
- Be aware of smells, dust, noise, etc. associated with the materials, which may restrict the patient's participation in the activity and lead to non-compliance and feelings of failure.
- Ensure that all materials are of good quality and that any copying, printing, transcriptions, are of the best possible quality. In this way, the professional is demonstrating how much the person's ideas and work are valued (Kennett et al 2004).
- People must choose for themselves their own materials, colours and layouts, in order to establish ownership of the piece.

- Give examples of what the finished object could be used for and explain that any items not required by the patient can be sold to others (in a hospice shop, for example).
- For people who cannot express themselves in words, either verbally or in writing, e.g. those with cognitive or sensory impairment, or for whom feelings are too painful to talk about, suggest an art activity, such as silk-scarf making, glass painting or small woodwork projects, into which the emotions can be poured as the object is created.
- Offer examples of verses that might be appropriate, ranging from simple lines to those with a deeper and emotive meaning. These can be found in books of verses available in card shops and in the works of poets such as Khalil Gibran (1991), or song lyrics collected together in an album for people to look at. Having some idea of what patients want to say means that the therapist can supply a variety of possible verses for them to use as they are, or adapt.
- In card making, people who are unable to read because of fatigue, poor concentration or sensory or cognitive problems can have verses read to them.
- Try to prepare ahead and pre-empt any possible problems. Levels of cognitive ability and consciousness may fluctuate over the course of the time. If, for example, people are using a book of verses to choose the most appropriate, suggest that they mark the pages with Post-it notes and write the name of the person that the verse is for on the paper. This will be helpful for people with memory difficulties, but also means that the professional can finish the card appropriately, if the patient becomes no longer able to participate.
- Leave some 'homework' that the patient might like to try, say in the evening, or over a weekend.
- Relatives and other visitors can help with information, such as clarifying dates for cards, supplying information and photographs for diaries or life stories.
- Whilst the process is the therapeutic element of creative activity in many other clinical areas, in palliative care, the finished article has as much relevance for its creator as its production. It must fulfil several objectives, and be the container for emotions such as love; asking for and giving forgiveness; the communication of unsaid words and feelings; or offering thanks.
- The patient must feel that it is 'fit for the purpose' – well made and perfect for the person who will receive it. It should be something that patients can feel proud of for themselves, and when sharing their creation with others. They need to feel confident that it will make a gift that is well received, both for its appropriateness and for the visual effect.
- People will derive a lot of pleasure in seeing the transcript of their poems or text.

99

'It's how I felt about it, but it looks like nothing when it's all just written down higgledy-piggledy with scores-out and bad spelling. You've made it look just right – just the way I felt it.' Cara was astonished and delighted when she saw the finished card, decorated with clipart that she had chosen on the computer. She wanted lots of copies to share with others.

Examples of art projects

- Silk painting can be used as a group activity, e.g. using a free-hand technique, long silk scarves can be flooded with colour from pipettes to create wall hangings. These can have a

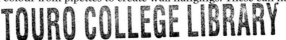

theme, such as depicting the elements, or be random explosions of colour. Individual activities can be graded according to abilities, and include scarf making, using the technique already described, to complicated pictures which can be mounted in cards or made into cushion covers, or framed.

- Glass painting is a versatile activity. It can be a small project, such as a sun catcher for a new conservatory, a child's room or decorating the window in the ward. Sheets of acetate can be coloured using specialist pens, giving the effect of stained glass, and then fitted into aperture cards. Acetates with adhesive backing are especially useful for group projects, where individuals can paint their own sections, before they are pieced together to form one large picture. The sections can be outlined with adhesive lead strips to give the appearance of a stained glass window. Small projects can be scanned into the computer and the design used to make cards that the artist can send to friends.

- Collage is a useful activity for people who feel that they are not artistic, as the forms are already created for them in magazines, newspapers, etc. This can be purely a leisure activity, done on a very small scale, as in card making, or as a larger project, either copying a photograph or creating a completely abstract design. Images can be used as metaphors, allowing the patient to work through the significant issues that they represent. Group work involving collage encourages interaction and involves the members sharing their ideas and their feelings about the images. This in turn will foster understanding and empathy between the group members, often stimulating discussion about other things unrelated to the original theme (Williams 2002). Individuals may use collage to depict their lives, their likes and loves, their dreams and ambitions. The process of telling their story in pictures, using cuttings and photographs, can be a cathartic experience, as they work through various issues from the past and create the story of who they were, and who they are.

- Pressed flowers. This can be a group activity, addressing the differing needs and abilities of the group – collecting flowers and leaves (maybe by people with cognitive impairment who want to walk outside), pressing them, and using them in creative art projects such as card making and collage.

- Art activities can be photographed, or scanned and printed into greetings cards, notelets, or calendars, to be given to relatives and friends.

- Recipes can be made into books, or put on to calendars, along with the name of the person who donated them, so that people still feel they are giving something to the group even if they cannot actively participate.

- The back page of cards can be printed with the artist's name, or the gift can have a card attached with the name on it. This is a way of acknowledging the value of their work and increasing self-esteem.

Writing

Creative writing is a cathartic experience for the patient, using metaphor to externalise feelings, moods and emotions, where love, guilt, anger and regret spill onto the paper as symbols (Jensen & Blair 1997), producing a feeling of relief that at last the words have been released. These words reveal the essence of that person and as such, may be perceived as reflecting the spiritual element of the person's being.

It is often difficult for people to say aloud all the things that they want to. Somehow it is easier to write them down. This might be because the words can be reworked time and again until they are acceptable to the writer, or that the communication does not need to be face to face. People can easily identify with this as a reason for not sharing their deepest feelings, and are relieved to discover that there is an alternative and acceptable way of communicating these thoughts.

The first card that the therapist helped a patient to make followed a conversation with a man who desperately wanted to tell his wife how much he loved and appreciated her. This was something he had never done and he was unsure how to go about it. He had argued with her that morning and said things that he now regretted.

He felt that to say the words would be difficult and was afraid of what the response might be – would she just laugh at him? The card was duly made with great care and taken home. On his next visit, the man reported that that evening, after she read the card, they were able to talk about the illness and cried together. He was so relieved that they had rediscovered a closeness and felt that they could now support each other in the weeks ahead.

It is important to establish the purpose of the activity at the beginning. Is this a purely personal piece of work, intended for the writer's eyes only? Is it to be shared with the group, e.g. poetry writing; or are the reminiscence stories offered as part of a group activity session for the pleasure of sharing and having these stories or poems acknowledged? Or, thirdly, is it to be given to someone as a communication of feelings and emotions, or legacy?

Some writers choose to destroy their work – it may have been enough just to externalise their feelings and share them with the therapist, and so nothing more needs to be done. The realisation that the business is no longer unfinished brings with it feelings of pleasure and relief.

Whatever the purpose of the written piece, the reason for its creation will have an influence on how it is developed and on the final outcome in terms of satisfaction that a particular concern has been dealt with.

Diaries

Diaries can be a record of personal and intimate thoughts, detailing the illness narrative, and providing an outlet for the maelstrom of emotions involved in that person's experience. This may be seen by the relatives as a memento of that person's last few weeks and days and can become a precious and lasting legacy. Diaries can also include photographs – of the person participating in activities, of patients with loved ones, such as sitting in the grounds in a favourite part of the garden, or Mum reading a story to her child, lying cuddled up on the hospice bed. Visits from pets can also be recorded in the diary in this way. Favourite flowers can be pressed and added to the pages, and artwork scanned or photographed, as described in Chapter 12.

Poetry

Poetry, as a style of creative writing, develops an image (Robinson 2004) using words, in the same way that artwork uses shapes and colours. These words are powerful, with metaphors and symbols used to depict unutterable thoughts and leading the way to completion and closure in certain areas of that individual's life story. People may use this activity to express their feelings about a situation, whether happy or sad; to record their feelings about changes or significant times in their lives; or perhaps to try to find an explanation for their dreams. They may choose to share these words with others, to help resolve strained relationships (Abiven 1995). They may feel that they can help others by sharing their experiences with them, sometimes personalising the poetry by using the name of the recipient in the verse, or by leaving their poems to others as a legacy or a way of saying goodbye.

A number of poems written over the period of the illness may be pieced together to form a journal, perhaps including poems written at other times in that person's life, and creating a different style of life story.

Written and visual images

These can be combined in several creative activities. Some people might like to include some of their work in the order of service for their funeral. This project will be as individual as the patients themselves and often takes the form of a style of life narrative, incorporating photographs, and verses and lyrics from favourite songs, intermingled with religious material such as hymns and readings. The images used may be a collage of the important stages of that person's life, illustrating the quintessential elements of a unique being.

> Penny always liked organising things – parties for friends, outings and surprises for the people she loved. She wanted to make sure that her memorial service would reflect how she had lived – happy, vibrant and enjoying the company of all of her friends. The order of service was planned to the last detail, including the colour of card, style of type and the picture of a beautiful rose for the front cover. A collage of photographs filled the inside of the cover and Penny wrote poems to be read to the congregation and chose the songs that were to be played. The very last page showed a photograph of her waving farewell and the whole thing was held together with a red ribbon to match the rose. A number of copies were made and stored in a shoebox in the staff duty room until Penny's friend collected it after her death. A member of staff who attended the service reported that Penny's friends had felt that it totally represented her.

Card making is perhaps the most popular way that people choose to express themselves using word and image.

Difficulties related to speaking the sentiments aloud can be bypassed as feelings are not expressed in the presence of the recipient, making the disclosure of these much easier. Writing, as a communication activity, allows for a retrospective appraisal of the situation, from both the writer's and the recipient's perspectives. It also means that words of support can be given, even after the patient's death.

> Lucy knew how nervous her daughter would be at exam time. She wanted to offer her the words that she needed to hear at that time. But the exams were next year and Lucy would not be there for her daughter. She made a beautiful card for her instead, offering all the words of encouragement that she thought Angela might need.

Life storybooks are a further example of using a variety of creative media and techniques together in one project. This activity serves several purposes – it not only recognises that person's achievements, but it is also a legacy, a collection of memories that the individual regarded as significant and wanted to share with future generations. Unlike verbal storytelling that can distort or fade over the years, these recorded memories are tangible and enduring.

People can do creative activities with their children and grandchildren. This can make the visit a positive experience for the children, and allow them to reflect on it favourably (Kennett et al

2004). The artwork can then be used in a memory album, recording the time spent together in the last weeks or days of life. This is described further in Chapter 12.

Ensuring success

Seeing examples of others' work, whether displayed in the activity room, or viewed in an album of ideas, will encourage patients to attempt activities, or join a group. People are delighted when they discover that their work can look just as good as that of others and they feel inspired to suggest other activities that they would like to try.

Careful monitoring of participants' abilities, and listening to their unfolding stories will ensure success and continued participation as they move from using creativity in a leisure sense to a more psychodynamic approach. Feeling comfortable and relaxed will give patients the confidence to begin to explore sensitive and perhaps difficult areas of their lives, and revisit certain situations and experiences. Through working alongside and sometimes with the patient, listening to narratives and using counselling skills alongside the creative process, the professional can create opportunities for these cathartic experiences to take place.

People who are driven to carry out certain creative activities are willing to rearrange visitors and other activities such as hairdressing, having a bath, etc. in order to participate. They will muster the energy to be able to continue with and finish important work, and inpatients often ask what they can do over a weekend in order to complete the project as quickly as possible.

Relatives are delighted that the patient can still be productive and enjoy things, and they have lasting positive memories of that experience (Kennett et al 2004). It will provide a topic for conversation and visitors may also find that they can be involved in the activity – bringing photographs from home, for example, helping to list things that people have loved during their lives, such as favourite flowers, foods, music, for life-story or memory albums. The positive response from relatives and friends to the gifts, cards, memory albums and other creative activities is very satisfying for the patient.

> Ellen: 'Friends were very emotional when I gave them their gifts and cards. I was surprised at how much people think of me. I didn't realise it before.'

Relatives will have something of the dead person that they can touch fondly as they reminisce, and patients, knowing that they will be remembered in this way, feel comforted. Often these tokens will be used, in whole or in part, at the funeral service, providing happy and comforting memories for those left behind.

For others

The potential benefits from participating in creative activities can be experienced by anyone, not just patients. They can provide a distraction from issues that can appear all-consuming, allowing 'time out' in order to gather personal resources and take stock before moving forward (Holder 2001).

Issues relating not only to professional practice, but also to areas of personal involvement and concern, such as those surrounding death and dying can be explored using creative activities. Professionals and carers can benefit from artwork and writing as a means of understanding and expressing themselves, and as tools for reflection. As a learning tool for health professionals, perhaps during a reflective session, participation in collage work can be used as a prompt to much wider and deeper interaction within the group than discussion alone can achieve (Williams 2002).

References

Abiven M 1995 The crisis of dying. European Journal of Palliative Care 2(1):29–32

Allied Health Professions Palliative Care Project Team 2004 Allied health professional services for cancer-related palliative care. An assessment of need. Online. Available: www.palliativecareglasgow.info/pages/ahpproj.asp

Boog K 2006 The use of creativity as a psychodynamic activity. In: Cooper J (ed) Occupational therapy in oncology and palliative care, 2nd edn. Wiley, Chichester

Brown R, McKenna HP 1999 Conceptual analysis of loneliness in dying patients. International Journal of Palliative Nursing 5(2):90–97

Bye R 1998 When clients are dying: occupational therapists' perspectives. Occupational Therapy Journal of Research 18(1):3–24

Cassidy S 1991 Terminal care. In: Watson M (ed) Cancer patient care: psychosocial treatment methods. BPS books, Cambridge, p 149

Chochinov H, Hack T, Hassard T et al 2005 Dignity therapy: a novel psychotherapeutic intervention for patients near the end of life. Journal of Clinical Oncology 23(24):5520–5525

Devlin B 2006 The art of healing and knowing in cancer and palliative care. International Journal of Palliative Nursing 12(1):16–19

Fisher M, Fitzsimmons M, Thorpe H et al 1997 Psychodynamic counselling in specialist palliative care. European Journal of Palliative Care 4(3):105–109

Gibran K 1991 The prophet. Pan Books, London

Holder V 2001 The use of creative activities within occupational therapy. Opinion piece. British Journal of Occupational Therapy 64(2):103–105

Holland A E 1984 Occupational therapy and day care for the terminally ill. Occupational Therapy 47:345–348

Howie L, Coulter M, Feldman S 2004 Crafting the self: older person's narratives of occupational identity. American Journal of Occupational Therapy 58(4):446–454

Jensen CM, Blair S E E 1997 Rhyme and reason: the relationship between creative writing and mental wellbeing. British Journal of Occupational Therapy 60(12):525–530

Kennett C, Harmer L, Tasker M 2004 Bringing the arts to the bedside. European Journal of Palliative Care 11(6):254–256

Nainis N, Paice J, Ratner J et al 2005 Relieving symptoms in cancer: innovative use of art therapy. Journal of Pain and Symptom Management 31(2):162–168

Obrian J 2001 Providing scope for creative growth in palliative care. European Journal of Palliative Care 8(4):163–165

Peloquin S M 1997 The spiritual depth of occupation: making worlds and making lives. American Journal of Occupational Therapy 51(3):167–168

Perrin T 2001 Don't despise the fluffy bunny: a reflection from practice. British Journal of Occupational Therapy 64(3):129–134

Rahman H 2000 Journey of providing care in hospice: perspectives of occupational therapists. Qualitative Health Research 10(6):806–818

Reynolds F, Prior S 2006 Creative adventures and flow in art-making: a qualitative study of women living with cancer. British Journal of Occupational Therapy 69(6):255–262

Robinson A 2004 A personal exploration of the power of poetry in palliative care, loss and bereavement. International Journal of Palliative Nursing 10(1):32–38

Thompson M, Blair S E E 1998 Creative arts in occupational therapy: ancient history or contemporary practice? Occupational Therapy International 5(1):49–65

Vrkljan B, Miller-Polgar J 2001 Meaning of occupational engagement in life-threatening illness: a qualitative pilot project. Canadian Journal of Occupational Therapy 68(4):237–246

Williams B 2002 Teaching through artwork in terminal care. European Journal of Palliative Care 9(1):34–36

Wright J 2004 Occupation and flow. In: Molineux M (ed) Occupation for occupational therapists. Blackwell Publishing, Oxford, p 67

Play and leisure

Claire Tester

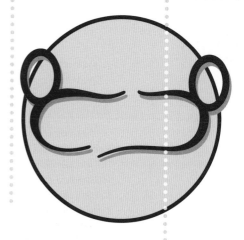

External as well as internal experiences can be rich for the adult, but for the child the riches are to be found chiefly in play and fantasy.

Winnicott (1964)

Key words

play; exploration; development; assessment; deterioration; senses

9

Play and leisure activities are to be enjoyed and are fundamentally creative activities. In palliative care with children, play is a valuable outlet for expression and channelling energy. It is a means of connecting and communicating with a child. Play can be used as therapy to maintain or develop new skills. In this chapter an overview will be given of the different aspects of play, the development of play into leisure pursuits and the importance of recreational activity for the adult, including the young adult. The difficulties in play with children with sensory impairment will be explored using assessment and different approaches with ideas and activities for parents. The emotional well-being of the child will be considered.

What is play?

Play is many things. When an adult talks of play it is understood to be a fun activity and light-hearted, for pleasure and enjoyment. In an adult world, play is perceived as a childish occupation and is simple. 'It's child's play' is used to describe the simplicity and ease of an adult task. Play when connected to a sport or a board game with rules and boundaries is seen as superior to the open-ended and imaginative play of young children.

However, play is serious and deeply important to a child and needs to be acknowledged as such. 'Play, which provides suitable opportunities to strengthen the body, improve the mind, develop the personality and acquire social competence, is therefore as necessary for a child as food, warmth and protective care' (Sheridan 1985).

Play engages the child totally and involves the emotions of a child. It is an outlet for expression, essentially creative (Winnicott 1964) and enables children to learn, explore, try things out, use the imagination (Sheridan 1985) and understand aspects of the world around them. This includes objects and their relation to each other, as well as people and emotions. There is excitement and tension included in child's play (Winnicott 1964). There can also be an element of anxiety which can be relieved through play as it can act as a channel for nervous energy. Aspects of repetitive or compulsive play may indicate a child's emotional state.

Piaget (1967) recognised that play was fundamental to a child's learning and assimilation of skills. Play has different developmental stages, each one a cumulative step from what has gone before. The development of play reflects a child's developmental age and stage of emotional development too. When working with a child it is necessary to understand the developmental stage of the child. The developmental stages or milestones are to be used as a guide. Children in palliative care are still developing and growing despite having a life-limiting condition. It is important to keep this developing aspect of the child in mind, for development needs nurturing and supporting even when for some children there is deterioration and loss of skills. Some conditions affect the development of a child and can cause regression, e.g. Sanfilippo.

> Mother: 'It's as if she's reached her full ability and is going backwards now. She only wants to sit and watch the same video of Teletubbies, hold the same toy and have cuddles. She is not interested in anything new nor any of her other toys.'

Types of play

There are different types of play. Each type is not a stage in itself but an aspect of a kind of play which continues to develop, reflecting a child's psychomotor development (Gassier 1984).

1. Active play – relates to movement; gross motor or large actions including the seemingly unfocused actions of arms and legs at infancy to the coordinated actions of mobility such as running, throwing, catching, etc.
2. Exploratory and manipulative play – beginning at infancy in taking hands to mouth as fists, through to coordinated fine motor and hand–eye coordination tasks.
3. Imitative play (from 7 months) – ranges from mimicking simple actions for a few seconds, such as opening the mouth in imitation of mother, to actions carried out independently, e.g. copying tasks. Such imitation involves coordination, sequential thinking and proprioceptive awareness.
4. Constructive play – from block stacking at 18 months onwards to model making etc., requiring gross and fine motor skills, sensory abilities and the ability to recall (Sheridan 1985) as there is an intention when building. The intention arises from a thought or memory held.
5. Make-believe or imaginative play – incorporating imitative play with imagination, e.g. washing dolls' tea cups to increasingly more sophisticated play creating scenarios with emotion and feeling.

6. Games with rules – from simple sharing of turn taking at toddler stage to developing cooperative play involving leadership, and fair play. This type of play extends to increasingly sophisticated team games and competition with formal acknowledged rules as in sport.

7. Recreational leisure pursuits – as individual or as a shared activity. These may include the development of a skill or activity which is lifelong and pleasurable.

It can be seen that there may be overlap between these different kinds of play and that they are not mutually exclusive. Play can develop into hobbies or leisure pursuits too. For example, a constructive activity requiring fine motor skills as a recreational activity such as embroidery or model making can become increasingly sophisticated into adulthood as a pursuit. Some of these activities may even be formalised such as in the Embroiderers Guild with group meetings, exhibitions of members' work and awards given for excellence. Even aspects of make-believe and imaginative play can be extended into adulthood appropriately, for example as drama and creative writing. As one actress remarked, 'I'm still playing make-believe, and dressing up. But it's in the theatre, and I love it!'

Play as therapy

Play can be used as therapy in two ways – as directive therapy or as non-directive therapy. Directive therapy is when there is a specific or stated aim to help a child maintain or develop a new skill such as balance, or an aspect of hand–eye coordination. The play is selected and directed to engage the child actively in the tasks in the playing. The setting may be anywhere, and others may be involved in the play. Such play is usually purposeful with an achieved or recognised end. It may be time-set by the therapist in relation to the child's level of concentration and attention, fatigue, when the task is completed as in a game, or by the adult's own availability. The time is not strictly limited. This is the most used form of play and is termed directive therapeutic play not play therapy. Paediatric occupational therapists use this form of play with children. A tension in different approaches can arise between the caring for a child, or person, and the therapy where an individual's response may take an effort. In therapy a child is encouraged to develop skills and abilities, which is not always understood by another health professional. For example, a therapist sat on the floor with a child on a mat. The child was positioned on his side to encourage his slight voluntary movement to effect a position of lying supine (on his back) as a play activity. A nurse accused the therapist of being unkind to the child.

Play therapy is a specialised non-directive form of therapeutic play and is carried out by a trained play therapist, child psychotherapist or paediatric occupational therapist with specialist training. This therapy uses a psychoanalytical approach and works at a deep emotional level with the child. A child is referred for play therapy. In order to establish security for the child there is a level of constancy in the setting and the time of a session. For example, the session is held at the same time every week for a set time (usually 40 minutes to 1 hour) at the same place with the same therapist and only the child. Toys and objects used in the setting are the same each week. The therapist provides skilled emotional containment for the child in order for the child to 'spill out' (Axline 1996) and also enables the child to work through emotional issues. The sessions are confidential between the child and the therapist, which is understood from the beginning. There are different play therapy approaches which cannot be explored here but are given as references for further reading. Children who are aware that they have a life-limiting condition or terminal illness can greatly benefit from play therapy. In this safe environment frightening and disturbing thoughts and feelings can find expression and understanding. This is emotionally painful work and the value of it is greatly underestimated.

Play specialists are able to select appropriate toys and playthings for a child in a hospital or hospice setting according to ability, and can help to reassure a child about to undergo an operation, etc. by redirecting the child's attention. Play specialists should not be confused with play therapists.

Sensory impairment

Children spontaneously play. But not all children have the same opportunities to play, for many different reasons. These can range from an inability to initiate play through sensory loss or developmental delay; through loss or deterioration of skills; because they are emotionally withdrawn or physically weak; or because opportunities for play are not given. However, all children need to be able to play, and the play needs to be taken to passive children and for them to be actively helped to engage with it. A common difficulty in selecting play items for a child is to use the age of the child as the determining factor for the stage of development and play the child would be capable of.

A boy of 9 years arrived at the hospice with story tapes and books to read in bed, and with toy cars. He showed no interest. On assessment, this little boy was low toned and unable to make gross motor movements without support, he was unable to focus but could perceive light and dark, and although he did not have any speech he could indicate when he was unhappy or pleased by crying or smiling. He was assessed by the paediatric OT as being developmentally at the 6 months stage. Consequently play ideas were centred around one-to-one interaction with the carer and on sensory activities. Play included being held and rocked with songs, being helped to explore his own hands by placing them in the midline on his chest with support, and being introduced to different textures which were placed in his hands and held with care to be taken to his mouth to feel and explore. Bath times and dressing were used as opportunities to use firm but gentle pressure, stroking the child's limbs to increase a sensory awareness of his own body. It was noticeable that the child was responsive and smiling. He was given a soft floppy toy dog which accompanied him throughout his stay and acted as a comforter for him. His sleep pattern noticeably improved.

Many of the life-limiting conditions of children include a developmental delay, as in mucopolysaccharide conditions; or neurological deterioration such as in leukodystrophy or Niemann–Pick disease; or are debilitating such as Duchenne muscular dystrophy. In cancer it is the site and progression of the cancer which may affect skills and sensory loss, besides the fatigue and weakness as side effects to chemotherapy. The emotional well-being of the child must always be considered. Depending upon age and intellectual ability, children may understand that they have a life-limiting or terminal condition and will die. Play can act as a means of expression and communication but requires a skilled practitioner to interpret and respond appropriately to the child.

Children with developmental delay and sensory impairment

Children who have a sensory impairment combined with an inability to initiate movement cannot explore their own self, objects, or their surroundings. They remain passive and are often unable to speak. Such children can present as difficult to play with, and activities can centre on watching television, or being taken out – essentially passive activities – in an effort to find something to do with the child. These children have so much to offer regarding play activities and sensory stimulation. As play is a form of communication with a child, a rewarding relationship can develop which is both exciting and moving. It can be difficult to know where to start in playing with a child who is sensorily impaired with a developmental delay.

> A nurse speaking of a 2-year-old child: ' Susan cannot speak, or move independently. She lies still and her mother says that she does not like to be touched. She is blind and deaf. She has a gastrostomy which she has had since birth.'
>
> This little girl, out of the five acknowledged senses of sight, sound, smell, taste and touch, appeared to have only smell to explore her outside world. But there were many things to help her connect with her surroundings and with others, through her other senses.

Working with a child who has a deteriorating condition and is sensorily impaired requires a careful assessment which gently explores a child's abilities to respond to different stimuli. These responses are described as 'skills'. In this way a child is regarded in a positive way as having abilities. Such an assessment helps to identify different ways of relating to the child, and helping others to relate to and understand the child. Assessment reviews help to identify how the condition is affecting the child's senses.

> Father said: 'My son doesn't like me any more, he doesn't look round when I come into the room.' He was upset, as his son used to look round to his father's voice and smile. His 14-year-old son was deaf and his vision was deteriorating, although the father was not aware of the degree and had been nurturing the idea over some weeks that his son was less interested in him and had decided to withdraw from his son, feeling rejected.

Assessments help to build a picture of the child. Sometimes medical notes can be scant regarding what the child is capable of and responds to, or when the child has deteriorated the notes may no longer be up to date. It is necessary to determine a baseline and to regard this as a positive beginning rather than an identification of skills the child lacks. Existing formal assessments involving task setting and motor skills performance cannot be used here as they are too challenging and identify what the child cannot do. They do not serve the child and can 'lose' the therapist. Developmental scales from early infancy to 5 years can be referred to (Sheridan 1985). When working with a child who may have more than one sense impaired and who is developmentally delayed, it has been helpful to assess using the senses as a baseline. It is generally accepted that there are five senses. These can be regarded as outward senses which respond to an external stimulus. For this assessment and to develop play ideas it is necessary to think of extending the list of senses to include proprioception, balance and motor-planning. These are core skills in sensory integration (Fisher et al 1991). Rudolf Steiner (Glas 1983) extended the senses to include sense of self as 'I' – the ego sense – as well as language sense and thinking sense, sense of warmth, and feeling – as expressed through the emotions, including a spiritual sense. This last sense may be outwardly expressed as an emotion of elation or happiness, which may be observable, though the cause may not be understood. However, it is helpful to bear a spiritual sense in mind when working with a child, young adult, or adult who is unable to communicate and has sensory impairment, for each person is unique and individual. A spiritual sense does not mean a religious faith or belief but can include it. This adds a further seven senses which can be seen as directed to an 'inner world' affecting the body and having a psychological effect (Aeppli 2003, Glas 1983, Soesman

2001). Assessment for some of these senses is explained at the end of the chapter, in Appendix 9.1. Working through the senses provides an opportunity to find different ways of connecting with an individual. Through the activities used in assessment, further ideas for play and communication present themselves to the therapist, and these can be developed and extended as therapy. It can be emotionally moving as connections are made. Time, patience, and a caring and sensitive approach with detailed observation skills are essential for the success of such an assessment. When writing, always emphasise the positive, and begin with it. This includes the appearance of a child. Using the language of the senses is more easily understood by parents and carers than using medical terms. Some of the activities in assessing lead easily to activities such as dressing and washing limbs, for example the proprioceptive sense which is also linked to the sense of touch.

Sensory activities

Using the sensory assessment enables one to identify ways to stimulate and engage with a person. For the child, parents can be encouraged to make different sensory boxes (from shoe boxes) collecting items for play. Each box has a sense theme, and items which stimulate a particular sense can be stored in the box. Suggestions include different items with a variety of textures, e.g. nail brush, flannel, sheepskin, wool, foil, sandpaper, etc. The box itself can be decorated and made into a colourful and tactile experience in itself. Sensory ideas as activities to stimulate the senses and to help connect with someone should be written simply for family members and carers to read, and the family should be encouraged to contribute ideas too. These ideas for activities are not prescriptive, or rigid. No-one's senses should ever be overstimulated, so a short burst of 15 minutes for taste and smell sense activities is long enough. Other senses such as touch can be explored for as long as an hour.

The adult who has sensory impairment

The adult who cannot communicate or appear to actively communicate can be assessed using these guidelines but not through 'play', as the approach needs to be sensitive to the dignity and age of the person. The responses may be identified in the same way but the objects and language used need to be appropriate. It should never be assumed that someone who cannot initiate movement or communicate actively is not capable of feeling or thinking. It is one of the challenges of the therapist to reach the person. Jean-Dominique Bauby (2004) had 'locked in' syndrome, dependent for all his needs, being able to only move his left eyelid. A therapist used a pointer stick and alphabet board, responding to his blink as assent for a letter. He indicated he wanted to write. He was a journalist. A secretary was employed and he wrote his autobiography in this way. He planned his words and paragraphs the night before and memorised them. They were then ready for the next day for typing. He was keen to let others know that he was aware of people speaking over him, and describing him as a 'vegetable'. It does not mean that all who cannot initiate movement are capable to the same degree as Bauby, but there should always be an awareness and respect of another's thoughts and feelings, and a real wish to connect with the person. It is possible to further isolate someone who has deteriorating skills and sensory impairment by attitude and ignorance. When a connection has been made with a person, no matter how slight, it can make so much difference when shared with the child or person's loved ones.

A mother communicating through gentle touch with her paralysed, blind and mute son who was losing his vision: 'I know that he knows it's me. I can feel him relax as I touch him. This is lovely. I feel I can talk to him in a different way,' she said tearfully.

A 10-year-old daughter, who was unable to initiate movement, blind and fully dependent for all needs, was losing her hearing. The mother was encouraged to talk to her daughter through the child's cranium at the temple points, and at the sternum, so that the child could associate the mother's sounds with vibration. The mother felt this gave her a feeling of hope that over time in her daughter's limited life she would be aware of her mother, and the mother could reassure her daughter in different ways, of which this was one, of her presence.

Sensory boxes for adults who have sensory impairment must be age appropriate and relevant. For example a hand massage for touch, combining favourite scented creams for the hands and feet. Favourite and personal smells, such as the husband's aftershave, or the person's own perfume, can arouse the sense of smell. Any aromatherapy massage oils should use a simple almond oil as carrier. It is helpful to check with a qualified aromatherapist regarding contraindications for some oils before using them. Children enjoy making and decorating these for a relative.

Leisure and social activities

As discussed earlier, an individual cultivates interests and hobbies, some with specific skill and knowledge acquisition through life. Such interests may have been formalised or may have remained informal and not clearly apparent. Enquiring about people's interests may be identifying a dimension of what has given meaning and purpose to their life. Therefore finding how these interests may be pursued when skills are being lost can be important to a person, and may contribute to a quality of life. Depending upon the degree of sensory and motor loss, one may need to be inventive. It is appealing to the senses which provides direction. As many activities include social activity and inclusion it may be that company is a substantive part of preferred activities. For example, to be able to attend a club's social event, or to visit an exhibition can mean a lot to a person. To identify what is meaningful to someone is fundamental (Frankl 1978). Young adults with life-limiting conditions will usually continue to attend school, perhaps on a part-time basis and may struggle to participate in social activities, both within and outside of school. It is necessary to support them to be as active as possible. Access to public amenities has improved, although it may still be necessary to telephone ahead, e.g. to the cinema or theatre, to ensure access. Social isolation as a person's condition deteriorates can be hard to bear. The social and emotional needs of an individual must be considered in addition to the physical needs.

Small equipment items such as forearm supports (attached to wheelchair), or different operating modems for computers and games consoles can enable some interests to be continued. As skills can be lost, continuous assessment is needed and equipment needs must be updated.

One young man had become noticeably withdrawn until it was discovered that he could no longer operate the joystick control for his computer, and was no longer emailing his friends, nor playing computer games. He admitted that he 'felt useless' and was 'good for nothing'. However, a different device was found which he could use and he did regain a positive sense of himself. It was only when someone asked the young man about himself and what he enjoyed doing that the difficulty came to light.

There are many technological devices available which are worth exploring. Specialist books may be available on tape or CD. Where there are activities involving a tactile and physical dimension, this could be introduced, e.g. to be able to handle items, models, etc. When people may not see or hear they are still able to gain from their other senses.

One young woman who loved horses was taken to a stables where the smells and sounds brought her obvious pleasure. As she deteriorated, a horse was brought on a visit to the hospice to her window. Her bed was taken to the opened window and her hand extended passively to touch the horse which nuzzled her hand. Her eyes flickered and her heart rate quickened.

Conclusion

Everyone is unique and individual with thoughts and feelings. In palliative care a child or person may have deteriorating skills and abilities, including impairment of the senses. The therapist has an important role in maintaining independence at all levels, and this involves a connection and communication with others. It is necessary to find out about the child or person's likes and dislikes, things that have been enjoyed in the past, from the relatives and loved ones. But more than this, it is important to link the person with an activity which has meaning and purpose for that individual, and brings real pleasure.

References

Aeppli W 2003 The care and development of the human senses. Steiner Fellowship, Sussex

Axline V 1996 Play therapy. Churchill Livingstone, London

Bauby J-D 2004 The diving bell and the butterfly. Harper-Collins, Canada

Fisher A G, Murray E A, Bundy A C 1991 Sensory integration – theory and practice. Davis, Philadelphia

Frankl V 1978 Man's search for meaning – an introduction to logotherapy. Hodder & Stoughton, London

Gassier J 1984 A guide to the psycho-motor development of the child. Churchill Livingstone, London

Glas N 1983 Conception, birth and early childhood. Anthroposophic Press, New York

Piaget J 1967 Six psychological studies. Random House, New York

Sheridan M 1985 Spontaneous play in early childhood. NFER-Nelson, London

Soesman A 2001 Our twelve senses – wellsprings of the soul. Hawthorn Press, London

Winnicott D W 1964 The child, the family and the outside world. Pelican, London, p 144

Suggested further reading

Bernstein G A, Kinlan J 1997 Summary of the practice parameters for the assessment and treatment of children and adolescents with anxiety disorder. Journal of the American Academy of Child and Adolescent Psychiatry 36(10 suppl): 69S–84S

Burke J 2005 A new approach to paediatric palliative care. Online. Available: http://www.ebility.com/articlles/bearcottage.php 30 Oct 2006

DeBord K 2006 Childhood years: ages six through twelve. Online. Available: http://www.ces.ncsu. edu/depts/fcs/human/pubs/child6_12.html 25 Oct 2006

Focusing on how people are motivated and make choices, utilise skills, the impact of the environment and how these affect the health of the individual. Adult and paediatric volitional assessments

Guide for playthings. Online. Available: http://www.sickkids.ca 2 Nov 2006

Huebner A 2000 Adolescent growth and development. Online. Available: http://ext.vt.edu/pubs/ family/350–850/350–850.html 2 Nov 2006

Hyun E 1998 Making sense of developmentally and culturally appropriate practice (DCAP) in early childhood education. Peter Lang, New York, ch 2. Online. Available: http://www.ruby.fgcu.edu/ courses/ehyun/10041/culture_and_development_in.htm 2 Sept 2006

Kielhofner G 2002 A model of human occupation – theory and application. Lippincott, Baltimore

Lewis M, Ramsay D 2004 Development of self-recognition, personal pronoun use, and pretend play during the second year. Child Development 75(6):1821–1831

National Association of Paediatric Occupational Therapists. Information on membership available from College of Occupational Therapy. Website: www.cot.org.uk

Play therapy – information on training, publications and members available from the British Association of Play Therapists. Online. Available: http://www.bapt.uk.com/professionalinfo.htm

Powell J, Smith C 2006 Developmental milestones: a guide for parents. National Network for Child Care. Online. Available: http://www.nncc.org/Child.Dev/mile1.html 3 Nov 2006

Sheridan M 1975 From birth to five years – children's developmental progress, 3rd edn. NFER-Nelson, London

Stages of play development in delayed children. Online. Available: http://www.braintraining.com/ PlayStages.htm 3 Nov 2006

Appendix 9.1
Sensory assessment

Claire Tester

The following guidelines for assessing senses and levels of communication in children, can be used with young adults and adults who may be described as sensorily impaired or in an unresponsive state. The items used must be age appropriate and not considered as toys which would be readily used with infants and children.

Assessing

The purpose of this assessment is to get to know the child, to reach out and connect with them. It should not be hurried, and the approach needs to be gentle and considerate. In many ways therapists can be considered as using all of *their* senses to find out about the child. It is presumed that the medical notes will be read and that the child's condition is understood. The therapist needs to observe the child initially, to identify movements to any stimulus, and any movement whether involuntary, reflexive or active. The position of the child, seated or lying, should also be noted, because it may make a difference. It is helpful to observe any interaction of the child with another – this could include while a pad is being changed, or medication is being administered. If a parent is carrying out any of these tasks, the child may respond differently to a well-known person rather than one who is less familiar. It will be necessary to find out amongst the staff those who consider themselves to have a relationship with the child and to find out more about their interaction.

When assessing it is better to be with the child in a quiet room which has natural light and curtains, and is private for the duration of the assessment. It will not be possible to assess each of the senses described in one session. A child must not be bombarded with too much stimulation. The assessment in itself can provide aspects of play which act as a form of cognitive stimulation. For small children and infants it is easier to have them lying on a bed or soft mattress with the head supported by a small pillow. Depending upon the child's degree of movement, the sides of the bed are placed in the 'up' position. Assemble objects you require before the session and have them out of sight. The suggestions below are given to assess some senses in a rudimentary way to inform ideas for play. They are not formal assessments and cannot replace formal assessments by optometrists or audiometry tests. Health visitors use standardised tests for developmental assessments too. The suggestions set out are to help assess a child or person with one or more sensory impairment and to provide a baseline for abilities. It is assumed that each sense will be assessed in a quiet room with the door closed and the child made comfortable. Another person may be in the room to assist, but must remain quiet. Make detailed notes during the assessment as you go along. It may be necessary to put a 'Do Not Disturb' sign on the door for the duration of your assessment, and also to inform others of what you are doing. Often a closed door of a child's room can be opened suddenly and the feeling of calm and quiet you have created for the assessment as well as the tentative responses a child or person has begun to make can be shattered. Time and patience are needed to carry out the tasks and to observe for minute reactions. Each aspect of the sense assessment is an attempted form of communication. They may not all 'get through', but occasionally they might and this can be very stimulating for all involved.

Sight

Here the assessment is based on determining what the child can see and if there is a restricted range of vision. A person may be described as being blind and unable to see but might be able to discern light and dark, or movement. When assessing sight do not use an object which has any sound or smell, e.g. a rattling toy. Sight needs to be assessed sensitively and thoughtfully. Observe the child or person in a day-lit room. Does the person look around, or follow the movement of someone across the room? Next try moving an object across the line of vision. It is important to keep yourself, or anyone else if being assisted, out of the line of vision, as the attention must be on the moving object. Move an object across the line of vision and observe the eye movement as well as any head movement. Use a brightly coloured object, ideally of one colour, which can be seen more clearly against a background. A patchwork object is harder to discern for someone with limited vision. Move the object closer until there is eye movement and a degree of focus. This may not occur.

Next darken the room and use a small torch or lit object. Again try moving it across the line of vision and watch the child's eyes intently. Observe any eye movement and reaction. Sometimes a child might show movement of the body as if excited. Do not give any verbal cues such as 'I am going to move this object in front of you', as from experience, the child may attempt to move the head and to cooperate when there is little or no vision.

Try moving the object at different speeds across the line of vision – moving something very slowly gives time for a reaction. Try different planes of vision, e.g. diagonal, vertical and horizontal. A reaction may occur that appears to be an involuntary motor movement. If this is the case, leave the exercise a few minutes and repeat it to see whether it was a coincidence or a reaction associated with the stimulus.

Sound

It is extremely important to have a quiet and enclosed area. Build up the degree of sound and sensitivity in the assessment. A first stage can involve a whisper near the child's ear. Observe constantly for reactions. When someone cannot initiate movement, a reaction might be seen in the eyes or facial features. It is helpful to have someone helping in the assessment who is either doing the whispering or observing and taking notes. Observed reactions can be small. It may be necessary to repeat actions too. Call the name of the person from the left side, and wait for a reaction for a minute. Repeat three times. Move closer and repeat the exercise. This can be done very close to the ear but not too loudly at this proximity. Then repeat from the right side. Use a xylophone or triangle to make single notes and let the sound reverberate near, but not right next to, the person. Occasionally a high-pitched musical note can receive a reaction that a voice cannot. Such a reaction can give rise to a form of musical communication with notes and made with pauses to wait for a reaction and another note sounded as in a conversation. Sounds in a hospital can be continuous background noise, which means that silence can provoke a response. A single sound or voice breaking this silence can be powerful. When assessing for responses to sound, silence is a good starting point.

Smell

Different smells are already present in the environment of the person and it is helpful to identify these first. Some of these smells will be associated with people, such as the perfume worn, and some smells are linked to procedures such as changing a pad, bathing or medical procedures. Some of these smells have either pleasant or unpleasant associations. Through observation, it is helpful to gauge whether there is any anticipation of an event. A usual link is when the smell of food arouses interest in a child or person. This does not apply when a child is tube fed; however, for someone who has a memory of eating, the smell of food can still arouse a reaction. Food items such as a cut lemon or chocolate, as well as spices with strong smells can be used. They are best used fresh and should be real rather than artificially simulated. Smells which are both attractive and repugnant are balanced to provoke an observable reaction. As smells can linger, it is not possible to assess using a whole range of smells in one assessment session. Also, too much olfactory stimulus may induce nausea, which should be avoided. Different smells can be used as a form of communication too, to help a person associate and anticipate specific people or actions/activities with certain smells.

Taste

This accompanies the sense of smell and as such can be assessed at the same time. For someone who is tube fed the sense of taste may be underdeveloped, as for example in a child who has been tube fed from birth, whereas for other children and adults a gastrostomy tube may have been introduced at a later stage when the person has a memory of taste. Taste can be assessed for a reaction by smearing a little of something on the lips, not food. This can be done with flavoured lip salve or, for example, with the merest hint of the foodstuff such as a little lemon juice applied to the lips. A reaction is often seen with the tongue exploring and licking the lips. Again, as in assessing for smells, a maximum of only two or three tastes should be introduced, as it can be too much stimulation. There is a reaction to preferred tastes and to rejected tastes. For example, lemon can cause a pursing of the lips and a reluctance to lick the lips after an initial exploration. A soft cloth for wiping needs to be kept to hand to clean the mouth. Experimenting with and exploring tastes and smells can be very enjoyable but care must be taken not to upset the child/person as it can be seen to be invasive. When applying anything to the lips the action needs to be gently explained beforehand, and rather than smearing the whole mouth area, care must be taken to apply the salve etc. gently and in stages; it should not be applied in one go. Be careful to observe any reactions or movements of the body as well as of the face.

Touch

A child or adult may initiate movement and reach out to touch. How the person touches involves fine motor movement coordination and sensorimotor ability. This can be assessed according to other assessments. In these guidelines, the quality of touch and awareness of touch is explored. When approaching a child or person who is unable to initiate movement and may not be able to hear or see, touch is the main indicator of your presence. When assessing for touch it needs to be considered in isolation. That is, when touching someone do not appeal to any other senses at the same time. Do not wear a perfume, make a sound, etc. when approaching the person. Try to touch those who have sight out of their range of vision. Touch needs to be appropriate and sensitive.

Initially touch the hand at the fingertips on one side, whilst observing for a reaction of the face, or of the hand itself or upper body. It is easier to assess one side of the body at a time as there can be variation at each side. If there is no reaction, then move to the dorsum of the hand and apply light but firm pressure with one's own hand. If there is no reaction, then hold the hand, applying palm-to-palm pressure. This also introduces a sense of warmth and of pulsation to the other person. With infants and children with small palms this pressure can be applied, but gently. Time needs to be given for the child or person to register what is happening and to make a response. This may take a few minutes. If there is no response, gently move to the wrist joint and hold it gently and firmly but in no way restrictively to apply pressure, and observe any response. Continue moving your palm in a single stroking motion along the skin on the medial (inside) aspect of the forearm where there is more sensitivity than on the dorsum of the arm. It is essential to be mindful of any drips or butterfly needles in the arm and any undue sensitivity from needle sites. At the shoulder, place your hand over the shoulder girdle and apply gentle pressure. Move gently to the side of the

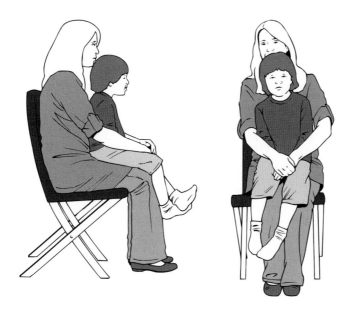

neck and rest your palm there. This is a sensitive area. If there is no response, then move in a stroking movement to the cheek. Repeat the process on the other side of the body. It is important for the approach to be gentle and slow, and sensitively used, observing throughout for reactions. Use your voice and touch as a response in reply.

Balance

Balance is assessed as a righting reflex and as sitting balance. This sense is assessed here when the individual cannot sit unsupported. This aspect of the assessment should be carried out only if safe to do so and with assistance. This is more difficult to assess for an adult or large young adult. For the infant or child it is necessary to sit with the child so that you are yourself in a fully supported position, and the child sits on your lap. The child leans back. If you hold this position for a few minutes, the child can feel the sensation of another's body warmth and heartbeat. This in itself can provoke a reaction which is physically felt by the therapist. Sometimes the heartbeat of the child can quicken.

The therapist supports the child with her body, bringing his arms into his lap, and with her arms applying gentle but constant pressure to his sides (see diagram). This provides a sense of physical safety for the child while being held.

Very gently and slowly the therapist sways to one side with the child. The therapist can physically sense any righting adjustment the child wishes to make. When this is sensed the therapist moves back to the centre position and waits several seconds before repeating the action on the other side. This gentle rocking motion acts as part of an assessment as well as enabling an element of therapy and play to be introduced. A gentle see-saw song can be sung, or, for a child, a game of 'going down and going up' can be played.

Exploring balance enables the introduction of balance to a child who would not normally receive the experience of balance and associated movement. Assessing balance with a young person or adult is not essential but can provide an opportunity for a parent or adult family member to hug and embrace the person and provide stimulation of gentle movement. It must be stressed that moving and handling equipment is necessary to hoist an adult and also that there needs to be a minimum of two other adults capable of assisting, and who can sit on either side. The person providing the 'hug' needs to be fully supported from behind, and should be at least as big and heavy as the person who is being helped to sit in a supported position. When sitting in this way, an adult does not sit on someone's lap as the child does, but between the supporting person's legs. Therefore the depth of seat needs to be big enough to accommodate this position.

Proprioception – sense of movement

This sense of movement is the perception of where the limbs and joints are in space, either when the body is static or during movement (Fisher et al 1991). It can be observed particularly during dressing and bathing.

In considering movement it is helpful to consider the movement which has been experienced by the child or adult in the past. 'For a little child the mere moving of his limbs is play enough at first' (von Heydebrand 1988). Some children with deteriorating conditions may have lost motor skills, and other children will not have had active movement at any stage. This should be considered as a part of the assessment. For example, one child who had been able to walk and had lost this ability in his deterioration, was fully supported in an overhead hoist which was lowered so that the soles of his feet were placed upon the floor. He showed awareness and pleasure through his facial expression.

During dressing and bathing, a child may be passive but may be able to indicate some muscular intention in putting arm into sleeve, stretching leg into trouser 'leg'. For children who have not had the opportunity or ability to explore their own body as infants, nor had the physical stimulation of being able to motor plan and coordinate their limbs (as in walking), then the way in which they are handled and touched is significant, and can be made more meaningful. For example, in bathing: 'I am going to wash your arm. Here is your elbow, down to your wrist and now your palm, and each of your fingers.' Then talk through each finger. This requires time and it is important too that when limbs are exposed the child is kept warm and is not in discomfort. Dressing provides the same opportunities. Children who are unable to initiate any movement in gravity often enjoy the passive movement of limbs in the water of a bath, jacuzzi or small pool when supported.

Warmth

Steiner (Aeppli 2003) describes this as the first developed sense. The sense of warmth is felt in the womb and when the baby is held in the mother's arms and against her body. Warmth is felt externally on the physical body and internally when full and content with milk. This warmth is aligned with nourishment and love. This aspect of warmth is in language, for example a person may be described as being 'warm' meaning caring. This contrasts with being 'left out in the cold' or a person being 'cold'. So the sense of warmth has different levels: physical, psychological and emotional. When assessing a child who cannot move or has sensory impairment it is helpful to remember that this is a basic and early sense. The response to being held, wrapped in a blanket or a warmed towel after bathing, can be readily witnessed as a physical relaxing of the body and as a secure sense of being held. The positioning is usually in a semi-fetal position. The regard and behaviour of the carer is as significant as the physical warmth and holding position. This sense of warmth and the required approach cannot be underestimated as it is simple but effective. Consider how as an adult needing some comfort, one might wrap the duvet around oneself in a sitting position with legs up. This sense is experienced as an awareness of nurturing in its different guises.

Feelings – emotions

This aspect is assessed in parallel with the other senses. The responses and reactions arising from working through the other senses inform the assessor of an emotional profile. This may be of reactions to aspects the child does not like, shown by withdrawing, turning the head, or facial grimacing. They provide a starting point from which to work and contribute to the profile of abilities to respond, and of likes and dislikes. Regarding a spiritual sense, this may not be possible to assess or determine, but it is helpful to consider it. It is aligned to love.

> A 15-year-old, unable to move actively, without speech, and with limited vision, was introduced to a piece of classical music. His facial expression could be described as one of elation and calm. Another example is of an 8-year-old girl, unable to initiate movement, without vision, with a gastrostomy, and to all intents passive. Her mother telephoned the hospice to check on her daughter. The phone was held to the child's ear and the mother was encouraged to talk to her child directly. The child remained silent for a couple of minutes, then, without any change in her facial expression, she began to make little sounds which were quick and small. Her heartbeat quickened. There was a recognition of her mother's voice and a need to communicate to her. This child had not been heard to make sounds before. The child's mother was not anticipating that her daughter would make sounds and was very moved, as were the staff who witnessed this.

This assessment is by no means thorough, nor is it standardised. Assessments for cognitive abilities exist for a far more detailed assessment, but are all linked to more able individuals. The intention is to provide an immediate baseline of abilities and to identify reactions and responses which may be very slight and easily missed. Such a baseline of skills and sensitivities can inform the approach used. For example, a young adult who was unable to initiate movement, was blind, and unable to speak, always became distressed in the shower. After the above assessment had been carried out, items for showering, such as flannel, shower gel, etc., were assembled and, before leaving her bedroom, they were introduced as touch and smell with explanations of being about to go into the shower. In the shower room the water was introduced to her hand, which was held outstretched first. This approach resulted in the young woman being relaxed and anticipating the shower. She was noted as calm and able to anticipate what was about to happen by associating the smells and flannel with the shower.

Sense of self

This relates to bodily senses as well as an ego sense. Steiner describes this as a 'sense of life' (Glas 1983, p. 86) as an inner comfort and contentment, directed inward to an inner world rather than a response to the outer world of the child. This can be observed by the sense of discomfort – a recognition of not being content and showing this whether through pain or hunger. This clearly links with the emotions and feelings being expressed when a child is unhappy, or in disquiet. The difference is that the child experiences this as from within rather than as a reaction to an external stimulus. It provokes the question, 'What's wrong?' An investigation begins: is it hunger, a dirty pad, an uncomfortable position, etc.? This sense of self can also be regarded as a choice of what the child does not want, what the child enjoys, or does not enjoy. This is a sign of the individual's will and feeling.

Assessing communication through the senses

This set of guidelines for assessment will only be used for children and individuals who cannot speak or communicate easily. Communication can take many different forms and should be extended into its widest sense of communicating through the senses. This may not be initiated by the child but is given as a response to the stimulation of a sense. This has a crossover with the demonstration of emotion and reaction but can also be a physical response which is a communication.

A child of 12 years, unable to initiate movement or to speak, and blind, was given a stroking massage when fully clothed. This involved a bilateral approach working down the upper and lower limbs with long stroking movements and gentle pressure at the joints. The child had been breathing quickly and showed signs of anxiety until the massage began. The movements were carried out in a slow and rhythmical manner. The child's breathing slowed and her muscle tone could be felt to relax.

This is an example of communication in a different way, without words, from the therapist to the child and in the child's response to the therapist.

References

Aeppli W 2003 The care and development of the human senses. Steiner Fellowship, Sussex

Fisher A G, Murray E A, Bundy A C 1991 Sensory integration – theory and practice. Davis, Philadelphia

Glas N 1983 Conception, birth and early childhood. Anthroposophic Press, New York

von Heydebrand C (1988) Childhood – a study of the growing child. Anthroposophic Press, New York, p 55

Using guided imagery as a relaxation technique for self-help

Kathryn Boog

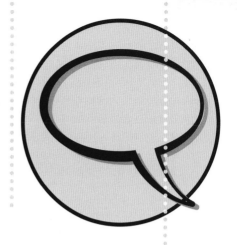

[Relaxation is] a valuable behavioural modification to help patients cope with the stress of disease and treatment.

Ahmedzai (1998)

Key words

self-help; control; non-pharmacological; symptom management; cultural considerations

Chapter contents

10

For those with a terminal diagnosis/prognosis, the complexity of their situation can be overwhelming, causing feelings of being powerless and leading to an increase in the severity of symptoms that may consequently prove difficult to alleviate. Despair and demoralisation may follow, further increasing their experience of pain, breathlessness, fatigue or other symptoms, until the whole situation seems to be spiralling out of control. People feel helpless, thoughts become muddled, and the whole process results in the person feeling disempowered, exhausted and unable to think clearly. The relationship between intensity of physical symptoms and levels of anxiety and distress is reported in the literature (Bruera et al 2000, Payne 2000, Strong 1991, Tanaka et al 2002) with relaxation advocated as a coping strategy to help reduce these (Ahmedzai 1998, Keable 1985, NCHPCS 2002). Similarly, it has been suggested that relaxation techniques are a useful self-administered method for dealing with nausea and vomiting resulting from chemotherapy (Redd 1982), and relaxation and imagery can significantly improve mood in patients undergoing radiotherapy for breast cancer (Bridge et al 1988).

Its aim is to encourage the body and mind to work together to develop a calmer state, in which thinking can become clearer, encouraging more logical and rational thoughts and helping the patient to regain some control, perhaps through its influence on the autonomic system (Payne 2000).

Guided imagery as a form of relaxation is a reliable coping strategy that can be used alongside pharmacological regimens, incorporating it into symptom and lifestyle management programmes. It is a simple and effective intervention that can be taught to people to enable them to assume responsibility for the management of their symptoms and to have some control over them. Those who are very weak or fatigued are still able to participate, as it is a passive activity and one that is easily transferable from the clinical area into the home situation. It is non-pharmacological and non-intrusive and can be incorporated into a person's lifestyle where increasing confidence in the value of the method as a coping mechanism enhances quality of life. The success of the intervention increases self-awareness and a belief in the ability to manage aspects of their life that have value and meaning for people. In this respect, it can address the spiritual elements of life.

Guided imagery can clear the mind and help the person to refocus by displacing negative thoughts and encouraging positive ones – producing feelings of increased energy and alertness. People can use their imagination to allow themselves to still do the things that are now impossible for them – such as running, climbing, walking or visiting a place that they love. The session can be structured or semi-structured according to need, making it versatile and adaptable, and it may also be cathartic, facilitating the expression of deeply held thoughts and the emotions related to these.

It is a method of relaxation in which participants are encouraged to actively use their imagination to create positive images that will induce a feeling of well-being and relaxation. Much is made of the use of the senses, for example picturing pleasant scenes or relaxing colours, and the arousal of the memories that particular senses evoke is used to create a positive mood. In guided imagery, these metaphors are introduced to act as a screen between patients and their unpleasant thoughts, minimising the influence of symptoms such as pain, and so allowing other, more acceptable and pleasurable sensations free rein. By using this coping skill, patients can gain some control over the management of their symptoms, resulting in a return of some independence and an improvement in self-esteem.

In everyday life, people use daydreaming to relax. This is an altered state of consciousness in which we de-stress, and takes place on average about every one and a half hours. It involves the right side of the brain, the area responsible for dreams and imagination, metaphor and symbolism and where emotions such as stress are processed. In guided imagery, the therapist is encouraging patients to use this right hemisphere to daydream and so reduce their levels of stress.

The technique can take several forms:

- It can be structured, as described above, where the facilitator describes the scene, encouraging the use of the senses to experience the imagery. By directing the participants to focus on uplifting and pleasant sensations and the moods evoked by these, a relaxed state can be encouraged, and practice will make the negative feelings easier to replace with the more acceptable, pleasurable ones.
- It can be semi-structured, where the facilitator will use the words 'maybe' and 'perhaps' in the script. A variety of scenarios are suggested, in order to stimulate the imagination, but leaving the patient to decide which to choose. This method can vary from being prescriptive to vague, depending on the patient's particular circumstances.
- Unguided visualisation allows even more freedom to use the imagination and is more empowering as it allows patients to be where they want to be in their imagination.

People usually progress at different rates from the structured to the unguided stage, depending on their imaginative abilities and how quickly they gain experience.

Narratives

The narratives/storylines used in guided imagery can be tailored to patients' individual needs, encouraging them to relive the mood of a particular positive experience, such as a visit to the countryside or being at home in their own living room with someone they love close to them and within earshot – somewhere they feel safe and comfortable. In order to create the appropriate mood, it is important to listen to the patient's personal narrative so that images that are meaningful to the patient can be used.

Assessment

During the initial assessment process, consideration needs to be given to:

- The reason for referral.
- The presenting problem and levels of tension/anxiety.
- Communication issues:
    - The patient's level of understanding.
    - Whether the patient has sensory impairments, e.g. a hearing difficulty. If so, consider using a Loop system.
    - Can the patient understand the language in which the session will be conducted? If not, is it possible to use a tape in the patient's preferred language?
- The subjective assessment – life story, illness narrative – information gathering and initial patient interview.
- The objective assessment – observation of the individual including body language, breathing, agitation/restlessness, dry mouth, distraction, fidgeting, legs crossed, arms crossed, drumming, watching others.
- The sensory experiences that you might introduce and their appropriateness – if people suffer from sweats and hot flushes, they might like to imagine a cool scene; if they have fluid retention they might want to imagine themselves light and floating instead of heavy and relaxed; be aware of the patient's body image, pain and fatigue levels and the issues that are causing them anxiety and distress.
- How much explanation will be needed.
- The patients' level of interest in learning the technique and their willingness and motivation to participate, as it is a form of self-help requiring commitment from the participants.

Observation

Throughout the relaxation session, careful observation of the patient will allow the therapist to adjust the script accordingly and to notice any behaviours that may need to be addressed either during the session or later. These might be one or more of the following:

- fidgeting
- tears

- jerky movements
- swallowing more
- sleep talking
- apparent discomfort
- agitation
- feeling uncomfortable and/or embarrassed
- irregular or distressed breathing
- changes in breathing pattern
- swollen limbs
- increasing signs of anxiety
- sleeping/snoring
- grimacing
- opening eyes.

It is important not to make particular people feel that they are being singled out, but if someone is drumming her fingers, for example, make general suggestions such as: '*You might feel that your shoulders are becoming looser . . . your elbows . . . your wrists . . . through your hands and into the joints of your fingers . . . your fingers feel as if they are getting longer . . . and looser . . . and more relaxed.*' If this is unsuccessful, you may need to approach the person and put your hand on her arm so as not to startle her, before asking quietly, '*What are you feeling, are you all right, would you like to talk about it at the end?*'

Signs of being deeply relaxed might be:

- jaw falling open
- head slipping to one side
- feet falling out to the sides
- shoulders dropping
- breathing slowing, becoming regular and less laboured.

At the end of the session

- Remind patients that they can go back to this relaxed and safe place any time they choose.
- Emphasise the importance of coming back gently out of the relaxed state and of getting up slowly. When people are deeply relaxed, their blood pressure falls and they need to be told to allow themselves time to become completely reorientated before attempting to move around.
- Some people like to continue relaxing with their eyes shut in order to prolong the pleasurable feelings or the memories and the mood that they have experienced.
- Discuss how relaxation can be included in the daily routine and how it fits into pacing and planning activities – suggest that it can be used before visitors arrive, before outings, or as an aid to resting during the day, but not sleeping, making it easier to sleep at night.
- Supply an information booklet and tape; encourage the use of the tape at home, as continued practice will allow the relaxing images to be recalled at the onset of anxiety, before it spirals out of control.
- Suggest that they can write down worrying thoughts before their relaxation time and put them on a table beside them or in a drawer, to be dealt with later.

- Emphasise the importance of using a quiet place, taking the phone off the hook, choosing a time when visitors or carers will not be calling, and involving others who can help to ensure that the relaxation can be practised undisturbed.
- Ask about progress at the next session and provide support, changing the imagery as appropriate, or encouraging the use of people's own images. Continued group work at the day hospice or visiting on the ward and offering the opportunity to repeat the session 'live' will also provide useful back-up and encourage people to continue.
- Encourage sharing this activity with their spouse or carer. Suggesting sharing the relaxation session at home with a spouse or carer in order that they too may benefit will often result in patients' acknowledgement that their carer is anxious or exhausted.
- Strongly advise against using the tape when driving.
- During the reorientation period at the end of the session, some may want to share their personal images with the group, which can then lead to a general discussion or sometimes to reminiscing.
- It can also take the form of a debriefing session where feelings may need to be discussed, either in the group or individually. The relaxed state will often lead to a release of emotion, which may be a great relief for some people, but for others it will lead to the unwanted externalising of feelings. This is discussed further under 'Considerations' below.

Contraindications

There are several contraindications to using this technique. These will be revealed at the assessment or at the introductory stage at the first session:

- Some people may only be able to focus on the negative – severely depressed individuals, for example.
- Anyone who is actively psychotic and who cannot therefore distinguish between reality and imagination or who experiences hallucinations or delusions, or confusional states is an unsuitable subject for this approach.
- Pain must be adequately controlled.
- Participants must have enough cognitive ability to understand the technique.
- Those who have difficulty creating images and using their imagination, will not be able to participate.
- It is not a suitable technique for those who are very distressed, and it is not a crisis intervention.
- People who take diuretics may not feel able to relax, especially if they are new to that particular treatment, as they can be preoccupied with toileting. Bowel problems may also make participation difficult.

Preparation

Offering a comprehensive explanation of the proceedings at the start of the session will encourage trust and confidence – building relationships which will allow people to participate more readily in the group and have more faith in the benefits of the technique, leading to a more successful outcome.

- Inform others who may be in the vicinity of the room that the patients are participating in a relaxation class as part of their treatment programme and that keeping noise to a minimum for the duration of that class would be much appreciated by the patients. Notices outside the room will act as a reminder.
- The room should be warm but not too hot or cold. Perhaps rugs may be needed. Explain to participants that they will be lying still for some time and may feel the cold more.
- There should be adequate ventilation, perhaps using fans.
- Suggest that people might want to go to the toilet, have a drink or take medicines beforehand.
- Make sure that people are comfortable – sitting, reclining or lying – and provide cushions or footstools as required.
- Introduce new members to the group and anyone who is joining in – students, staff, etc.
- Ensure that the Loop system is set up and working, if it is being used.
- Each time new members join the group, explain the principles of relaxation, what will happen during the session, how long it will be (20 minutes is a good length of time), how they might feel at the end. This may also be appropriate to refresh memories from time to time.
- Use stories as examples to show how the method has worked for others and thus how it might work for these participants.
- Give people permission to 'switch off' from all external stimuli – say that the therapist will attend to these. Encouraging a trusting relationship will allow people to acknowledge, but not feel that they have to respond to, a whole selection of external disturbances. Even fire alarms will seemingly be ignored.
- Encourage people also to acknowledge any thoughts that pop into their head and then to try to tune in to the therapist's voice again.
- Explain that relaxation is something that needs to be learned and that it may be difficult to begin with, but offer reassurance that after a few sessions it will be much easier. Improvement for patients happens in degrees and the more mastery they have over the technique, the more they will feel in control of their symptoms.
- Give people permission to move around in their chairs, cough or sneeze, as necessary.
- Check that the music and the presentation will be suitable for the whole group. Certain music may be distressing, evoking unpleasant memories. Using a familiar tune may also result in the person focusing on that and what is coming next, rather on the imagery. For these reasons it is often advisable to use New Age music rather than perhaps a classical piece which is recognisable to patients.
- Ask people which imagery they would like you to use. Individuals who constantly ask for the same one may want to be given the opportunity to talk about the meaning it has for them.
- Explain that you will tell people when to become aware of their surroundings and stretch and open their eyes, but ask if anyone would like to be left relaxing or to fall asleep at the end of the session. Tell those who wish to do so that they can, and to rouse themselves when they are ready.

Technique

- Make yourself comfortable.
- Use some passive physiological relaxation first, followed by the imagery of choice. Talk about the body sinking into the cushions of the chair, or being supported by the mattress, then

relate this to the idea of sinking against the sand on a beach or lying on soft, springy grass in a garden. '*As you experience these lovely feelings of relaxation, be aware of your jaw loosening and slackening, your shoulders beginning to sink deeper against the cushion . . . etc.*'

- Suggest that they are breathing in all the comfort around them and breathing out the anxiety and tension: '*Breathe in the comfort . . . and out . . . the anxiety . . . just let it go . . . out into the room . . . and away . . .*'
- It may be appropriate to discuss breathing exercises for dealing with anxiety and panic attacks, followed by the relaxation. Examples of these can be found in Appendix 10.1.
- Be alert to the response you are receiving and adjust your delivery accordingly. The patient's out breath is their relaxing breath so try to work with them. If working with an individual, it is possible to time the in/out of the waves on a beach in your script, with the person's breathing pattern, gradually slowing it down.
- Take your time. Introduce ideas and sensations smoothly – make linguistic links – the tendency at the beginning is to rush to get it over with.
- Use a script – it helps to keep continuity and flow, especially to begin with.
- Try to keep your voice soft and even. Lower your voice as you progress and allow it to deepen and slow down. Make the pauses longer as you progress. This is evocative of people's altered state of consciousness, as they become more and more relaxed.
- Evoke different senses in order to reach everyone – sight, sound, taste, smell, touch. People vary in which sense is predominant in their imagination.
- Feel that you are experiencing the things you are describing in real time – give your group time to become absorbed in their experience. You cannot expect to tell people that they are walking across a meadow to a tall tree in the distance and in the next breath that they have reached it. If you suggest people might be taking off their shoes and socks before walking in the rippling waves, give them time to do it!
- To rouse people – raise your voice, tell them to bring themselves back to the room and to be aware of the noises going on around them. If they are deeply relaxed, you might need to touch them or use their name. Tell those who want to that they can continue relaxing for a short time longer.
- Sit with the group until they become fully alert, as this is the time when discussion often occurs.

Feedback at the end of the session can throw some light on existential issues, cultural influences and what holds meaning for the individual, helping in the selection of appropriate treatment programmes and activities for that person. When they are in a relaxed state people can experience a rush of emotion that can be welcome, bringing with it happy memories and a desire to share these with others. They may want to continue the mood for longer by talking about their experiences and telling their own stories. Recall of uplifting memories that hold meaning and purpose for the individual will assist in the recognition and re-establishment of self-identity and personhood.

However, these feelings can also be upsetting and unwanted – letting go of guilt, anger and resentment or frustration can bring tears and embarrassment, and if not dealt with appropriately may lead to the person opting out of future sessions. This cathartic release of emotion can occur during the session or afterwards, and an appropriate response might be: '*I can see you are upset. Sometimes when you are relaxed, these thoughts come into your head – it's just because you are so relaxed. We can talk about it at the end of the session if you would like to.*' This is a situation when counselling skills can be useful, but it is important to recognise your limitations and to seek the involvement of another member of the multidisciplinary team (such as the clinical psychologist) for further support. Some people may find the process too introspective and choose not to continue.

If a tape is used instead of the facilitator being present, the opportunity for the distressing event to be explored may be missed, resulting in further distress, not only for the patient, but also for others in the group who may have witnessed it.

Considerations

- Recognise that relaxation is a powerful tool and understand your own limitations/experience.
- Experience the method yourself before starting to use it with others. This is necessary to be able to teach the technique effectively.
- Practise technique, timing, etc. by yourself at first. If you talk about walking over to something, do it in your head and then you will know that the others have reached there too.
- Delegate if it is appropriate and you are convinced that the person has had adequate training and will be aware of issues arising during a session.
- When introducing physiological relaxation methods at the beginning of the session, remember that people all naturally breathe at different rates and so in a group situation the dialogue must be couched in such a way that people can choose their own pattern. Also, for those with dyspnoea due to their illness, particular breathing exercises are neither possible nor desirable as patients may not feel comfortable with them and it may be physically impossible for them to comply, leading to distress. Passive methods are more appropriate before a guided imagery relaxation session.
- The imagery should have meaning for all of the participants in the group. Where this is not possible, individual sessions will be more appropriate.
- Be aware of using images that people find upsetting – some people have a fear of water, birds, sand, darkness, etc.
- Some people have a dread of relaxing and letting go, as they feel they will no longer be in control, or that if they lose control, they might die. (This is similar to when people do not want to allow themselves to sleep, or insist that they cannot be left alone.) It can be recognised by restlessness, perspiring, trembling, and rapid breathing, and may lead to panic attacks. These people may choose to opt out of a session.
- Although guided imagery is an activity that requires participation in order for it to be effective, patients do fall asleep on occasion. This is actively discouraged in most areas, but in palliative care, people who are able to escape from stress in the relaxation session should be allowed to continue sleeping if they wish (Fanning 1988).
- Remember that, as with all interventions, guided imagery will not work for everyone.

Scripts

The dialogue must be appropriate for the cultural needs of the group members. This will involve listening to people's stories in relation to their life narrative – roles, relationships, values and experiences. People must be able to relate to the images being suggested and feel comfortable with them in order to be able to participate in the session. For people whose first language is not English, it may be possible to obtain relaxation tapes from local cultural groups or ethnic libraries. However, it is still possible for those who are unable to understand much of the language used to benefit from the session, as the tones and modalities of the voice will have a soothing and relaxing effect, supported by the music.

There are several styles of imagery that can be used. Each dialogue is followed by about 15 minutes of music, before the participants are encouraged to rouse themselves, using the method described above.

- Metaphor – Participants, in the relaxed state, listen to the story unfold whilst identifying with the subject of the story. This frees them from the limitations of their own existence and allows them to do things that they cannot otherwise do. In the first example in Appendix 10.2, people can behave as if they are autumn leaves and detach themselves from their base, floating above the world and experiencing/seeing things from a different perspective. They may feel that they are distancing themselves from their situation (Payne 2000).
- Guided imagery – The description of the scene will contain elements of all of the senses, encouraging the person to concentrate on pleasant sensations, and creating a particular mood that will be influenced by the individual's unique slant on the imagery.
- Colours of the rainbow – can be used in the dialogue, with suggestions of how people might feel as each colour washes over them.

Examples of scripts can be found in Appendix 10.2.

Leaflet and tape

The tape, which is supplied for use at home, should follow the pattern of the relaxation session within the clinical situation. This will make it easier for the patient to identify with the principles of guided imagery as discussed at the first session. It should also last for the same length of time – 20 minutes. However, in order that patients may use the tape when they feel they would like to be able to fall asleep after the session at home, say, during the night, the reverse side should not include the dialogue that is used to rouse the patient, and the music should continue and fade out.

An explanatory leaflet should be provided, illustrating the key points of relaxing at home using the tape. An example of a leaflet can be found in Appendix 10.3.

For those who have difficulty imagining pictures, there are videos and DVDs available of relaxing images such as waves washing on the shore, or clouds drifting across the sky. Some have natural sounds whilst others are set to music.

Using guided imagery with children

Guided imagery can be used successfully with children and young adults. It can be in the form of a story for younger children that can be interactive, or for management of a specific symptom. An example of this relates to temperature control.

A young woman was experiencing discomfort at feeling so hot and was becoming overwhelmed by her body's inability to maintain any temperature control, so the therapist introduced the idea of guided imagery. The scenario for the script was discussed and planned together, as the South Pole. A vivid description of the frozen landscape and its features, including the howling wind and difficulty in keeping warm, was given. This image was carried by the young woman through the night. The next day she explained to the therapist that she had become extremely cold, and had had to send herself off to a hot beach in Florida to warm up.

Pictures, sound effects and sensory activities can be utilised as part of an enjoyable activity.

References

Ahmedzai S 1998 Palliation of respiratory symptoms. In: Doyle D, Hanks G W C, MacDonald N (eds) The Oxford textbook of palliative medicine, 2nd edn. Oxford University Press, Oxford

Bridge L R, Benson P, Pietroni P C et al 1988 Relaxation and imagery in the treatment of breast cancer. British Medical Journal 297(6657):1169–1172

Bruera E, Schmitz B, Pither J et al 2000 The frequency and correlated of dyspnoea in patients with advanced cancer. Journal of Pain and Symptom Management 19(5):357–362

Fanning P 1988 Visualization for change. New Harbinger, Oakland, CA

Keable D 1985 Relaxation training techniques – a review. Part two: how effective is relaxation training? British Journal of Occupational Therapy 48(7):201–204

National Council for Hospice and Palliative Care Services (NCHPCS) 2002 Fulfilling lives. Rehabilitation in palliative care. NCHPCS, London

Payne R A 2000 Relaxation techniques. A practical handbook for the healthcare professional. Churchill Livingstone, London

Redd W A 1982 Behavioural interventions in cancer treatment – controlling aversion reactions to chemotherapy. Journal of Consultant Clinical Psychology 50:1018

Strong J 1991 Relaxation training in chronic pain. British Journal of Occupational Therapy 54(6):216–218

Tanaka K, Akechi T, Okuyama T et al 2002 Factors correlated with dyspnoea in advanced lung cancer patients: organic causes and what else? Journal of Pain and Symptom Management 23(6):490–500

Appendix 10.1
Breathing exercise for anxiety-related breathlessness

Kathryn Boog

When people are anxious, the unpleasant feelings that they experience can be exacerbated by breathing too much. Taking in less air for a while will help to relieve these feelings. A useful exercise to help bring the breathing rate under control and to help people feel more calm is:

1. Focus on some inanimate object – a vase, a piece of fluff on the carpet – and concentrate on that.
2. Count whilst you are breathing. Say into yourself, not aloud, 'one thousand' whilst breathing in and 'two thousand' whilst breathing out.
3. Once you feel in control, try taking longer for each breath by counting 'one thousand, two thousand' as you breath in and 'three thousand, four thousand' as you breathe out.
4. Gaining confidence by practising this exercise whilst you are feeling calm, will allow you to start using it immediately you are aware of the anxiety starting, making it more effective.

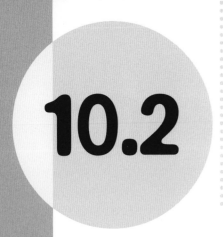

Appendix 10.2
Scripts for relaxation

Kathryn Boog

The autumn leaf

Imagine that you are an autumn leaf attached to a strong branch high in a tree in a forest.

All summer long you have basked in the sunshine and danced on the gentle breeze – a beautiful shiny green leaf reflecting the hot summer sun.

Now the cool autumn air has gradually changed your colour through yellows and oranges to a warm red, and it's time for you to be set free from your branch and to fly in the air, free as a bird.

As you swirl and dance in the cool frosty air, you cross wide fields and forests of pines.

Far below you can see the ducks gathering on a pond before they start their long flight south for the winter. You can hear them calling to each other across the water.

Every now and then you drift lower towards little farm cottages with smoke rising from the chimneys into the darkening sky. Inside looks cosy and bright.

Now the breeze begins to calm, and you drift gently to the ground and come to rest in a beautiful garden.

High above you the stars are shining and the moon is bright and clear in the frosty sky.

In the distance you can hear a little stream gurgling over some pebbles.

You are enjoying relaxing after your long flight, listening to the water washing over the stones, smelling the wood smoke from the chimney.

You are warm and comfortable in your little corner of the garden, relaxed and content and allowing your mind to drift with the music.

The fireside

Imagine that you are sitting in a lovely comfy chair by your fireside. The cushions of your chair are filled with soft, downy feathers, supporting you and allowing your muscles to relax.

You are surrounded by your favourite things – photos, ornaments, pictures, and the scent from the flowers in the vase smells so sweet.

It's a winter's afternoon and the lamps are switched on, giving the room a lovely warm glow.

Beside you, the fire crackles as some of the coals shift and settle, and you feel yourself sinking into the cushions of your favourite chair.

You can still taste the marshmallows you were toasting earlier in front of the fire.

Outside the streetlights have just come on and the orange light is shining on the frosty garden, where the children are laughing and playing in the fading light.

In the distance you can hear the music on the radio and the sounds of someone busy in the kitchen, filling the kettle and making the tea.

Your chair feels so comfortable, the cushions are so soft, supporting your body, helping you to feel relaxed. Your legs feel heavy, your arms feel heavy, and that heaviness is helping you to let go of the last bit of tension. Just let it sink into the cushions and away.

And as the tension goes, you feel so relaxed, your body feels lighter, and you allow yourself to drift along with the music.

A rainbow relaxation

Imagine that you are beside the sea on a beautiful coral island.

You are lying on the soft sandy beach and the palm trees are shading you from the hot tropical sun.

You can feel the gentle breeze stroking your face and your hair, as you lie there, relaxed and supported by the soft white sand.

In the distance, hear the sound of the waves as they wash in and out, in and out on the edge of the shore.

As you gaze out to sea, towards the horizon, you can see a rainbow high in the sky.

The colours are bright and vivid and they begin to drift towards you, bathing you in their light.

Feel the warmth of the red as it washes over you, and as you breathe, the warmth of the red spreads through you, giving you energy.

Gradually the red fades to a soft pink. Breathe this beautiful gentle colour into your body, right down to your toes, and feel yourself relax. As you breathe out, let go of any tension that you might have.

Now the pink light is fading to orange. With each breath that you take, let go of any worries and allow yourself to feel calm and relaxed. As your body relaxes, let your mind slow down too.

The orange changes now into yellow, the colour of sunshine. As the colour washes over you, you begin to feel calm, and at ease with yourself.

And now you are bathed in the green, the colour of healing. As you breathe, feel the healing mist flowing into your body, and reaching any part of you that feels uncomfortable – leaving you feeling happy and content.

The blue mist feels cool and relaxing. Any tension in your body is replaced by a deep sense of peace and tranquillity, and with the purple, you can let go of the last tensions and worries. Just let them go, carried away on the breeze.

As you continue to bathe in the wonderful colours of the rainbow, relaxed and content, listen to the music.

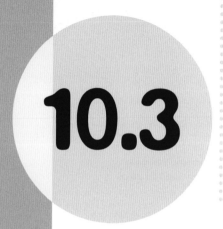

Appendix 10.3
Leaflet for relaxation

Kathryn Boog

Most people consider that watching television, reading or some sort of hobby is relaxing. However, whilst these are absorbing and pleasurable, they do not allow you to relax completely, as your mind is still working hard to think things through.

To completely relax, as well as resting our bodies we need to be able to switch off from all the thoughts that are swimming around in our heads.

The type of relaxation that you have been practising today is a way to do that. It is called guided imagery. This method can be compared to daydreaming, which we normally do at various times throughout the day – it is our de-stressing time.

On the tape, I will describe a peaceful and soothing scene, encouraging you to use your imagination. By focusing on this picture in your mind you should with practice be able to achieve total relaxation and finish the session refreshed and relaxed.

Before you begin:

- Make sure that you have been to the toilet.
- Find somewhere quiet – without radio or TV. Let your friends know if you do relaxation at a certain time so that they don't ring you at that time.
- Make yourself comfortable – do you need a cushion or a footstool?
- Don't let yourself be too hot or too cold.
- Give yourself permission to 'switch off' from all the noises around you.
- Acknowledge any thoughts that 'pop' into your head or sounds that you hear and then try to tune into the voice on the tape again.

And at the end of the session:

- Remember to stretch gently and to sit up slowly before taking a few moments to adjust to being fully alert.
- Take your time standing up.

Remember:

- Practice makes perfect. Relaxation is a technique that needs to be learned. You might find it difficult at the beginning but with practice it will become much easier.
- Practising the breathing exercise and the relaxation technique may allow you some control over certain worries and anxieties.
- It is important to pace yourself, building relaxation sessions into your daily routine. Planning your day, with times set aside for relaxation, may help with feelings of breathlessness and fatigue.
- Share your relaxation with your carers – let them enjoy the benefits too.
- Do not use this tape when driving.

Telling tales – the importance of narrative in our lives

Kathryn Boog

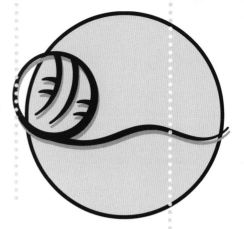

As we listen to a narrative unfold, we need to attune our ears to other stories buried within.

Linda Finlay

Key words

status; dignity; reasoning, meaning and values; the illness experience; psychodynamics; reminiscence; catharsis

Chapter contents

11

The use of narrative, as in storytelling, is a powerful and evocative way of enhancing our understanding of our world and our interactions within it. Past events are reflected on, assessed, reframed and re-evaluated against a background of the mood of the time, allowing for the formation of a comprehensive picture of these particular experiences. It is a reasoning process, where thoughts are organised and connections made between different memories in order to justify actions and make sense of them, thereby offering explanations for the choices that have been made. By examining these stories retrospectively, we have the added advantage of hindsight, which allows us to see things from a new and different viewpoint, helping to explain our behaviours and change our perceptions of them.

These narratives can be either internalised, where we muse, daydream or reminisce, or they can be externalised and shared. The telling of our personal stories is a subjective process in which we create our own identities within a cultural context, using stories not only to make sense of personal experiences, but also to demonstrate our unique roles and to gain approval from our peers, determining our sense of belonging and so enhancing our self-esteem. Viewing our lives in terms of successes and failures will reflect our estimates of our own worth and is a means of determining our status – how we are perceived and judged by others – and stories will evolve and change over time as we endeavour to achieve acceptance of our actions, both for ourselves and those around us.

The use of storytelling to demonstrate not only our own personal history, but also our place within our culture, is not a new concept. Cave art depicts the exploits of our ancestors; oral history has long been a primary method of communication for passing on tradition; rituals played out in dances and theatre portray the values of the past; the indigenous peoples of today still widely use metaphor to explain where they have come from, and who they are, for example by using the spoken word or perhaps tattooing their bodies with their own pictorial history to demonstrate their standing amongst their peers. These stories are legacies passed down through the generations, assuring continuity of ourselves for the future.

This desire for acknowledgement of status assumes even greater importance when we are confronted by challenges in our lives, and during periods of transition and crisis such as deteriorating physical and mental ability and impending death, when the search for meaning gains increasing momentum. There has been growing recognition in the last few years of the value of this type of reflection in reaffirming the dying person's unique sense of identity, worth and accomplishments (Wholihan 1992) and its place in the provision of dignity – conserving care (Chochinov et al 2005).

> Brian, a 59-year-old man with a history of alcohol abuse reluctantly attended the day hospice over a period of several weeks. During that time, he made no attempt to interact with other patients, although he would readily have conversations with the staff, sitting in another room and avoiding all social contact. He enjoyed talking about his past, a time when he had had many friends at the local bar where he was renowned for his storytelling and his quick wit. However, now that he was virtually housebound, these people had melted away leaving him feeling lonely and useless, resulting in low self-esteem and a poor self-image. During the course of many conversations, he revealed that not only did he enjoy storytelling, but that he had been known as a poet and used to give the vote of thanks, using limericks, at various gatherings he had attended. He was encouraged to take up writing his poetry again, and found great solace in being able to put his feelings about his situation into words. This progressed to verses read aloud to celebrate various occasions, such as at the end of the day hospice Christmas party, or following an outing planned by the staff, and he progressed to writing stories in verse about the day-to-day happenings in the day hospice. The others in the group greeted these verses with great enthusiasm and his rediscovered skill assured him of his status within the group as the person who would offer thanks on their behalf. The others began to sit with him and share stories and some asked for his help in writing verses of their own.

Revisiting the past has long been seen as a natural precursor to the end of life, associated mainly with the elderly, but its validity as a tool to enhance interactions with palliative care patients, across the age range, has been progressively gaining acceptance (Brady 1999, Chochinov et al 2005, Lester 2005, Lichter et al 1993, Pickrel 1989, Trueman & Parker 2004, Wholihan 1992). By finding out who people really are and what has been important in their lives, the narrative approach provides the opportunity to observe and be involved in the psychosocial processes involved in the act of dying – what is influencing that process for this person. The particular values and beliefs, including the spiritual, cultural and ethnic aspects, and the effect of these influences on the individual's life roles will help in the development of a holistic picture of this person.

In telling their life stories, or specific aspects of them, individuals have the means to confirm and understand the reasoning behind past behaviours, integrating these stories into the present, and providing a basis for moving on to the stories of the future. Situations that are perceived as having had a negative outcome can be revisited, reviewed and reworked and, whilst this process might not change things, it can allow the situation to be seen by the storyteller from a different, more acceptable perspective and allow the person to move on.

Whilst the life story will certainly offer an indication of how a variety of situations have been dealt with in that person's lifetime, these do not necessarily reflect how the person will respond to the stark realisation of impending death. Dying is a unique experience in the life of the individual. Although people may reflect on previous successful coping strategies in order to try to exercise some influence over the present, stress and losses related to dying are different, and people's inability to manage what is happening to them, by using these strategies, will only add to their feelings of powerlessness.

There may be factors from the past that patients need help with – unresolved issues that can influence coping strategies and colour their perception of their illness, affecting their ability to cope with the present situation and making management of symptoms more difficult. The complexity of these symptoms is identified widely in the literature (NHS QiS Best Practice Statement 2004, NICE 2004, Rahman 2000, SIGN 2000) and they manifest themselves in a variety of ways. Patients can avoid addressing the real issues that are making their illness difficult to manage by focusing on physical symptoms such as pain, as it is easier for patients and those around them to link their discomfort and distress to a physical problem, rather than to unresolved emotions. This, however, may result in a variety of stress-related problems such as nausea, vomiting, palpitations, breathlessness, feeling faint, panic attacks, etc. which do not respond readily to treatment (Lichter 1991). To be able to offer support in the management of these symptoms, we need to develop a wider understanding of their nature, searching beyond the medical notes and the physical disabilities, and into the real person.

John was sad and anxious on his arrival at the day hospice. His pain appeared to be uncontrolled and he regularly moaned and clutched at his chest, much to the consternation of the others in the group. He was unable even to eat lunch with his fellow patients and used pain as his excuse for non-participation in most activities, including conforming to a lifestyle management programme. The relaxation session was his only exception to this and in fact he relaxed extremely well, with no indication of pain during that time. He enjoyed these sessions and realised that they were a means of having some control over his pain. This was the basis for the formation of a trusting relationship between John and the therapist and led to the disclosure of the real reason for his pain.

John had always been head of the household, the breadwinner, the decision maker and definitely the person in charge. Since his illness, he had lost all of these roles. His status was changed and he had resorted to the sick role, pivoting his day around the routines of his medication. Communication with his wife had never been good, but now it was almost non-existent. He felt that the only time he could get any attention from her was when he moaned in pain. This information allowed the therapist to plan a programme for John to give him back some control in his life, to boost his confidence and his self-esteem, by teaching him how to prioritise, plan and pace his activities, and by suggesting ways that he could find a role for himself again and so deal with his relationship issues.

The psychodynamic life narrative (Burton 1991), where a counselling approach is used to listen to feelings and reflect them back to the patient, allows the meaning of that illness experience to be viewed in the context of the patient's life story. Peloquin (1997) compares this to looking at a stereogram – an image which at first appears to be no more than repeats of brightly coloured geometric designs. However, on closer inspection, and by looking past the design and into and beyond it, three-dimensional images are revealed. A holistic assessment, using narrative enquiry, can uncover the multiple facets of a life, furnishing us with a wider picture of the individual, leading to a deeper understanding of the person and the person's situation.

Entering into personal life stories allows the professional to see behind the illness to the real people – where they have come from, who and what they are – and is important in engendering an understanding of the impact of each illness experience on everyone involved. These stories evolve and change over time, influenced by changing circumstances and the reasons for narrating them. The storytellers redefine and modify the stories to make them more acceptable to themselves or their peers – perhaps in order to give meaning to the illness experience, or in telling them to a new social group (Clouston 2003). They are, however, the truth as perceived by the storyteller, and will be as individual as the narrators themselves.

Personal resources can be so compromised in the terminally ill, that patients feel that they are no longer capable of achievement. Demonstrating the positives, no matter how small, in a person's life, can help avoid any further lowering of self-esteem.

Diaries

Using diaries or journal keeping to record narratives can be a useful intervention in this situation. These diaries can provide useful information in the management of difficult symptoms, revealing underlying issues that are influencing the patient's perception of the situation, such as lack of self-esteem and relationship issues.

To begin with, patients may need help to complete their diary, as they may be so despondent that they feel they have nothing worth recording, and in this case, staff or relatives can help by offering examples and recording these in the diary.

> Walter was an ex-navy man, used to being in control of his life. He felt useless and demoralised and unable to see any positives in his daily life. He agreed reluctantly to keep a diary, recording his activities and making comments on how he felt. After only a few days, he was able to see that he was eating and sleeping better, and enjoying activities and some social contact in the day hospice. He was pleased that he had learned new creative activities and discovered that he had things to talk about with his visitors.

There are myriad styles of diary pages and an example is shown in Appendix 12.1. This can be easily adapted to suit individual needs. A further example used with a patient with learning difficulties is shown in Appendix 12.2.

Writing

As well as revealing their innermost selves to the listener, people can use narrative as a means of externalising their thoughts and fears, their dreams and hopes. Psychodynamic activity in the form of writing prose, poems, letters and cards allows people to record themes, stories and changes in their lives. Encouragement to use an activity such as poetry writing as a means of self-expression, can be a liberating experience, allowing the individual to work through feelings and to grow and move on. Seeing these very private things on paper somehow makes them more real and gives them credence, and they can be written and rewritten until they are acceptable to the author.

Judy had been having very vivid dreams – not frightening; on the contrary they made her feel reassured and content. She wanted to share the experience with her husband, but had always forgotten the dreams' content by the time he visited. Judy was encouraged to write her poetry describing the feelings she had about her dreams and she found this surprisingly easy to do, despite having never tried any writing before. She wanted them illustrated, and worked together with the therapist, at the computer, to find clip art that best depicted the themes.

Recording memories

Activities involving narrative can consist of words only, pictures only – using photographs and other images – or a mixture of both, perhaps including newspaper cuttings or magazine articles for instance. They may involve writing letters that will never be sent, or consist of a series of poems relating the life story of an individual, and can be pieced together to form a journal.

Eric wanted to share his memories of their relationship with his wife. They had had a wonderful time together and had never spent one night apart. Even now they were together, as both had a terminal illness and were inpatients at the hospice. Cerebral involvement meant that she was cognitively impaired, but he knew from her smiles when he was reminiscing that she still felt the same after all these years. He asked his family to bring in his boxes of photos, which he searched through, and proudly showed his favourites to the therapist, sharing stories and giving brief glimpses of the past. Together they worked to produce a memory album, mainly of photos, which Eric shared lovingly with his wife. 'And do you know,' he proudly announced. 'My mother-in-law said it would never last!'

The telling of the story alone, may be enough, but some people want to have a record of their lives to leave behind as a legacy for their relatives and friends. This album of memories and musings can be as large or as small as the individual wants and can be developed creatively in the same way as described for the memory album in Chapter 12.

Thoughts and feelings that are difficult to express verbally can be written in narrative form, whilst an order of service for the funeral can be a style of life narrative using words and photographs. These are described in greater detail in Chapter 8.

Relationships

Listening to people's stories and understanding why particular activities have meaning for them, gives us insight into their relationships and the role of previous occupations within these. Diminishing physical resources coupled with an imposed re-evaluation of hopes and dreams for the future can unsettle the individual's beliefs in personal values and goals. By using counselling skills during the interaction, in conjunction with an empathic relationship, patients will be encouraged to reveal how their life's meaning has been influenced by their changing life trajectory. The holistic view gained in this way will enable a supportive situation where both parties can work together to search out new and achievable goals which are both client-centred and realistic, and which will focus on improving and maintaining self-esteem and personal integrity and effecting closure on a practical, emotional or spiritual plane. This may involve working out how to deal with issues that patients feel remain unresolved or unfinished, or in assuring themselves that they will be remembered in a positive way. Personal relationships are one of the issues that often demand attention at this time, as past problems that patients felt had been dealt with at the time, can re-emerge with great and overwhelming force, influencing other factors in the management of the situation and leading to feelings of being out of control. Creative interventions can be used in this situation to facilitate communication with significant people in the patient's life, and these are discussed in Chapter 8.

Life stories

Where patients have very limited resources, making any form of physical activity unachievable, we need to help them change the emphasis of their view of themselves from that of a 'doing' person to one of a 'being' (Kissane et al 2001). To help in this process, relating narratives of significant events in their life should be considered as a positive and meaningful exercise (Lichter et al 1993), allowing patients to make choices about which stories to tell and how to tell them, and so encouraging the promotion of controlled self-expression. Where fatigue makes writing impossible for patients, they can choose to dictate the stories as and when their energy levels will allow, with the professional acting as the writing hand, providing a conduit for the flow of these thoughts and feelings.

The rediscovery of accomplishments and pleasures that may have been masked by subsequent negative episodes in that life leads to positive self-validation and improved self-esteem.

Philip wanted to make a doll's house for his granddaughter, but he had no time and extremely little energy to do this. He wanted to do something that would make her proud of him. Talking to him, the therapist discovered that he had been the driver of a steam train that rescued the passengers on another locomotive caught up in a landslide. She suggested that he could tell that story in a little album to let his grandchildren know that he had been famous and brave. A search of the local newspaper archive uncovered photos and a report, which were included, making a very happy granddad and an excited and proud little girl, who took her album into school to show her friends.

Relaxation

Previous pleasures in life can also be revisited in the form of images from the past recreated in the course of a relaxation session using guided imagery. Through listening to people's individual stories, it is possible to describe images to develop a favourite scene and recreate a particular mood. By describing the sights, smells, sounds, tastes, and tactile stimulation experienced in a given situation, such as walking barefoot across a field on a summer day or sitting beside a crackling fire in the early evening in winter, the person is encouraged to relive the feelings and sensations of a positive experience. Often at the end of the session, people like to share their particular memory with others in the group, which allows them to continue the mood for a while longer. This may then develop into a reminiscence session as others recall their own memories around the same theme.

Storytelling and group work can have a very positive influence on the quality of life of someone with terminal illness. Listening to people recount how they have dealt with past situations will allow professionals to suggest coping strategies to others in a similar situation, whilst for patients, telling their stories and hearing how others have dealt with their problems can be a supportive, and for some, a relieving experience, as comparisons are made and similarities drawn. Often just sharing the story once is therapy enough, but for some, the important aspect of it all is being given the opportunity to tell the story over and over again.

Reminiscence

Reminiscence is a social exchange and often relates to the recreational aspects of a person's life – events are generally discussed in a group in order to capture an emotional atmosphere or mood, and the feeling surrounding the memory is sometimes remembered more clearly than the event itself. It is considered an informal activity focusing mainly on positives from the past, but may evolve into the more formal and individual life review process where negative issues are reflected on, requiring a different approach. This is discussed in Chapter 7.

Reminiscence is a valuable group activity in palliative care for the following reasons:

- It enables participants to establish and re-establish their identity as a person and not as an illness, resulting in a feeling of continuity (of previous roles, status) and an affirmation of their sense of self (Howie et al 2004).
- Sharing stories can be a cathartic experience, encouraging and enhancing emotional well-being through a sense of belonging and integration into the group. Acceptance by others and the resulting feelings of connectedness will help counteract any sense of isolation.
- Feedback provides mutual support.
- People may feel that their lives have been dull and unremarkable. Having their own stories listened to and accepted by the others in the group immediately acknowledges their value, and knowing that others want to hear these stories gives the tellers pleasure and improves their self-esteem, thereby enriching their lives.
- Listening to others' stories may help patients to deal with similar problems that they themselves encounter, putting them into perspective and allowing them to be seen differently.

Individual reminiscing allows people to:

- Reflect on their whole life, choosing specific areas to reflect on: telling stories from childhood – about themselves, their place in the family structure, the part they played (in outings, significant occasions) up to, and including, the present. This theme is developed in Chapter 12.
- Work individually, using culturally appropriate props such as handling boxes.
- Go home at the end of the session and begin to think – internalising ideas and wanting to share more stories when they return.
- Just be themselves – to 'be' and not to 'do'.

> 'In the moment of delight, we are; . . .'
>
> (Verena Kast 1991, quoted in Byock 2004)

When using reminiscence as an activity, as with any other type of group intervention, consideration should be given to the following:

- Limit the size of the group so that everyone can have a chance to speak and allow for cohesion of the members. An intimate group will also promote an atmosphere of trust and confidentiality, allowing people to feel confident when sharing personal memories.
- There should be at least one facilitator per two to three patients. More help will be needed if recording stories or if patients require interventions on a more individual basis, e.g. those with cognitive impairments or sensory deficits, or people who have difficulty handling objects or concentrating for any length of time. Decide beforehand, with all of the facilitators, who will work with whom and the objectives of the session.
- Inform the patients of the theme on the previous week so that they have time to think about their stories and can arrange for visitors to the inpatient unit to change their visiting time if necessary. Fliers to take home will act as reminders.
- Discuss with members of the multidisciplinary team to establish who would be best suited to this type of activity.
- Plan ahead with other staff to lessen the chance of interruption, or patients having to make the choice between participation in the group and having a bath or their hair done.
- Make sure the room is warm but not too hot, the lighting is adequate, and props are readily available.
- Have patients organised in time – allow them time to go to the toilet, take medication, get comfortable – cushions, footstools, etc.
- Find out whether some people will be in bed, and make sure that there will be enough room.
- Ensure there will be no interruptions from noise or people. Once the group has started, no one else should join in, as this disrupts concentration and the continuity of the group.
- Discuss and negotiate with the other staff, including the hairdresser, nurses, volunteers, etc. Use a room exclusively for the reminiscence session and hang signs outside it.
- Ensure that patients are fit enough and still willing to join the group – fatigue, pain, breathlessness and anxieties about a variety of things may affect concentration and make participation difficult.
- People will be exposing aspects of their lives and may feel vulnerable doing this – it is necessary to make them feel safe.
- Participants may cry during the session – from joy, or perhaps from relief at finding someone to share particular thoughts with. This will need to be addressed and this is discussed in Chapter 7.
- Be aware of those who may unexpectedly have unpleasant memories, and be prepared to deal with that situation (as described in Ch. 7).
- Ensure that people have had their medication.
- Start and end on time so that people have the opportunity to do the other things they want to do. They will feel uncomfortable if they have to watch the clock and need to excuse themselves before the end of the session. Be prepared to shorten the session if this seems appropriate.
- Bring people back to the present.
- End on a positive note.
- Thank people for their participation and, if stories have been transcribed, ensure that everyone knows what will happen with their story.

What resources would be useful to act as triggers?
- Consider the different senses – touch, smell, taste, hearing, sight. Stimulation of these can encourage memories to flow more easily, allowing stories to develop.
- Music is a useful means of encouraging conversation. Compilations can be made up and used for 'Name that tune', using themes from films and radio or television programmes, or people

can be asked to bring in their favourite tune and talk about why they like it. If the group leaders are first to play their piece of music and discuss it, others will be encouraged to take part. Commercially produced tapes with sounds from the past are also available.

- Conversation during baking and cooking groups can be directed towards reminiscence, with the activity acting as the prompt.
- Use a common theme if trying to involve new members in a previously established social group. Start with a common denominator – although stories may not be from exactly the same time, they will relate to a shared theme. Use work, going out at the weekend – the theatre, cinema, dance halls – school, children's games, Christmas, birthdays, weddings, leisure, wartime, fashions. Consider cultural issues in relation to the content – is it appropriate? Some people from culturally diverse backgrounds might prefer to reminisce on an individual basis with the facilitator, using materials from their own past – handling boxes with appropriate contents may be available from local history projects, or cultural groups.
- A table displaying memorabilia collected from junk shops and charity shops will provide a focal point and arouse interest.
- Handling boxes, often available from local museums and containing objects from normal daily activities from the past, will stimulate conversation.
- Ask participants if they would like to bring in an object that has a story attached, which they would like to share with the group.
- Use pin boards and include themed photos and related stories from previous patients, books and magazines, online and local archives. Invite the participants to add their stories to those already displayed. Individual stories can be transcribed and enlarged and added to the display boards, or made into booklet form, to be read by others in the future.
- Transcribing stories to add to the display will improve self-esteem, as people realise that their memories will be shared with others over a period of time, not only underlining their involvement with the present group, but also connecting them to others in the future. They may be keen to participate in developing a booklet of stories that others who have not been involved in its production, might read. People will perhaps go off at tangents and want to tell their own story. This would be an appropriate opportunity to find out if they would like to work individually to develop a life-story book or memory album. For some people, the relaxed atmosphere of the session, coupled with the feeling of trust in the fellow storytellers, may result in individuals finding themselves talking about something that they have kept hidden over the years. The opportunity to share painful memories could be a cathartic situation for them, but it could equally be distressing or embarrassing. The facilitator needs to be alert to the group dynamic, and sensitive to the cues that indicate that a participant has unwittingly got into a difficult situation, or has more to say but not in the group context. The reaction of the other group members must also be considered, as some may not want to hear the story, but are unable to remove themselves from the situation. This would be an appropriate time to talk quietly and privately to the patient and introduce the idea of life review as an individual activity and is one of the reasons that it is important to have adequate numbers of helpers, who can maintain continuity with the rest of the group whilst the one-to-one interaction is happening.

Narrative for the therapist

Listening to patients' narratives, then, can enhance the understanding of who each person is and how illness has impacted on that person's lifestyle. This will allow realistic and achievable goals to be set, and ensure that interventions will be truly client-centred and the outcomes meaningful, representing the ethos of palliative care – that is, encompassing the physical, psychological, social, emotional and spiritual dimensions (WHO 2005). Using narratives to give examples of how useful others have found a technique can instil optimism and help combat demoralisation.

The effectiveness of the narrative approach relies on a number of elements in the interaction between the individuals concerned, a major prerequisite being the quality of the therapeutic relationship, which in turn is influenced by the personal narrative of the professional. This is fully explored in Chapter 1.

A narrative approach in the work situation may include writing a reflective diary – a tangible method of 'talking through' a particular scenario. Using narrative with ourselves, we can try out, or test, the dialogue we are considering, for example for a new intervention. Presenting case studies or narratives of client work (Bond 2002) is another practical use of this approach. At lectures and supervisory sessions, people become more interactive when narrative is used to demonstrate particular situations, perhaps because the listeners can link the story with their own practice.

The different elements of the patients' narrative are mirrored in those of the professional interacting with them. Everyone carries the accumulated baggage of life with them, and the influence of that baggage will reflect on the choices made – Will we open the box? Will our patients allow us to? And what will we do with the information?

Children and young people

Children and young people have stories too and can benefit from telling them. For children and young people there can be two stories: from diagnosis to the present; and the story of their life and family before this time. These two stories can be dramatically different.

For children, making a story book with photographs of family and earlier stages is often taken up by parents as a purposeful activity. This provides an opportunity to talk about past happier events, and to chronicle the life of a child. It is introduced as a story book for younger children, and as a photo album for older children to include friends and family. The way it is introduced, and the individual's own thoughts can vary; as one 12-year-old remarked, 'I'm not planning to die yet so I don't want a memory book thanks.'

Diaries can act as a narrative and can provide an opportunity for the affected child or young person to write intimately, as well as siblings. When diaries are given or suggested, it is important to discuss this carefully with the young person, recognising that there may be difficult things to write down, and upsetting things too. These things can be talked over with parents, or as a health professional you can offer support and an ear, providing an accessible work contact number to use. Thinking about children and young people in hospitals and hospices, it can seem as if everyone else is writing about them, and monitoring them. When even urine is measured and monitored, and bathing and toileting are assisted, there can be little privacy. As one 13-year-old girl exclaimed when given a diary, 'At last something for me to write in, and it's private!'

References

Bond T 2002 Naked narrative: real research? Counselling and Psychotherapy Research 2(2):133–138

Brady E M 1999 Stories at the hour of our death. Home Healthcare Nurse 17(3): 177–180

Burton M V 1991 Counselling in routine care: a client-centred approach. In: Watson M (ed) Cancer patient care: psychosocial treatment methods. BPS Books, Cambridge, p 82

Byock I 2004 The four things that matter most. Free Press, New York, p 104

Chochinov H, Hack T, Hassard T et al 2005 Dignity therapy: a novel psychotherapeutic intervention for patients near the end of life. Journal of Clinical Oncology 23(24):5520–5525

Clouston T 2003 Narrative methods: talk, listening and representation. British Journal of Occupational Therapy 66(4):136–142

Howie L, Coulter M, Feldman S 2004 Crafting the self: older person's narratives of occupational identity. American Journal of Occupational Therapy 58(4):446–454

Kissane D W, Clarke DM, Street AF 2001 Demoralization syndrome – a relevant psychiatric diagnosis for palliative care. Journal of Palliative Care 17(1):12–21

Lester J 2005 Life review with the terminally ill – narrative therapies. In: Firth P, Luff G, Oliviere D (eds) Loss, change and bereavement in palliative care. Open University Press, England

Lichter I 1991 Some psychological causes of distress in the terminally ill. Palliative Medicine 5:138–146

Lichter I, Mooney J, Boyd M 1993 Biography as therapy. Palliative Medicine 7:133–137

National Institute for Clinical Excellence (NICE) 2004 Improving supportive and palliative care for adults with cancer. NHS guidance on cancer services. NICE, London

NHS Quality Improvement Scotland 2004 The management of pain in patients with cancer. Best Practice Statement. NHS QIS, Edinburgh

Peloquin S M 1997 The spiritual depth of occupation: making worlds and making lives. American Journal of Occupational Therapy 51(3):167–168

Pickrel J 1989 'Tell me your story': using life review in counselling the terminally ill. Death Studies 13:127–135

Rahman H 2000 Journey of providing care in hospice: perspectives of occupational therapists. Qualitative Health Research 10(6):806–818

Scottish Intercollegiate Guideline Network (SIGN) 2000 Control of pain in patients with cancer. (Guideline no. 44) SIGN, Edinburgh

Trueman I, Parker J 2004 Life review in palliative care. European Journal of Palliative Care 11(6):249–253

Wholihan D 1992 The value of reminiscence in hospice care. American Journal of Hospice and Palliative Care 9:33–35

World Health Organization 2005 Definition of palliative care. Online. Available: http://www.who.int/cancer/palliative/definition/en/

Communication – making connections

Kathryn Boog

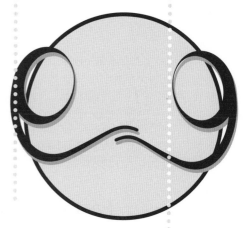

People's emotional responses to terminal illness can determine whether they live actively and positively, maintaining a hopeful outlook, or whether they are consumed with fear of what is happening to them or have anxieties about the future.

Jean Lugton

Key words

connections; cognitive and sensory issues; communication charts; assistive devices; creativity; memory making

12

The experience of terminal illness is multifactorial, and patients need to be able to share their concerns in order to work through certain issues and regain some equilibrium in their lives. People are complex entities, carrying with them all the baggage of their past (Lichter 1991), and the influence of these experiences will reflect on their present situation and affect the quality of their future life. Spiritual beliefs may be questioned, and people can feel demoralised by what they feel is a hopeless situation.

If this time is to be used for people to rediscover themselves, and to improve and maintain their perception of themselves and their lives, any concerns need to be expressed and people need to have the means to do this (CSBS 2002). They need to make connections – with themselves, with professionals (Ellenberg 2004), and with significant people in their lives, both past and present, and start to look at personal relationships and to concentrate on what matters – what gives their life meaning. This does not always have to be about issues causing emotional upheaval, but may just be stories that patients feel they want to pass on to others, to consider what certain experiences have meant, and to share them again with the people who were involved at the time. Perhaps this will involve telling others how much they are loved, or how proud their parents were and still are of them, or sharing memories of significant events from the past.

In reviewing their lives, people search for the positive contributions that they have made in the hope that they will be remembered in a meaningful way. Negative aspects will undoubtedly arise and people may want to take this opportunity to resolve strained relationships and make amends for past actions, or perhaps forgive someone else's behaviour, thereby finding closure (Abiven 1995).

Factors contributing to poor communication

Poor communication will inhibit these activities and may be due to a number of factors, such as guilt, fear, regret or anger, or simply not knowing how or where to start. These issues may be related to past actions, or to the present where patients may feel that it is their fault for being ill and letting others down. Improved communication will help strengthen interpersonal relationships, allowing people to discuss their feelings, to make choices and to have some control over the outcome of particular situations.

Terminal restlessness will also inhibit meaningful interaction at a time when communication is important, and may be due to physical, psychosocial or spiritual distress, complicated by fluctuating levels of consciousness. Good communication before this stage is reached will uncover possible triggers and allow a chance to work through these issues before they pose problems (Head 2005).

Compromised cognitive abilities and difficulties with articulation that result in an inability to use the spoken or written word will further compound the problem, as will times when the language used by patient and carer is different. People who are very ill may revert to their native tongue, although they may not have used it outside of the family for years, and using family members or friends to interpret is not always the best solution, nor is it in everyone's best interests.

Sensory impairments such as hearing and sight difficulties will cause barriers to good communication, and solutions should be considered, in order to facilitate the best possible interactions. Assistive equipment, such as LooP systems for people with certain hearing problems, advice on magnifying sheets and lighting for those with sight problems, adaptation of switches for nurse call systems and the provision of individually developed communication charts and diaries will encourage and facilitate a better level of communication.

> Steve could not understand why he suffered pain, nausea, anxiety and breathlessness. He was a poor historian and, although staff were sure his symptoms were due to overeating, he was unable to comprehend this. It was decided to ask him to record certain information in a diary and because his reading and writing skills were very poor, pictures were used. He was asked to put a tick in the boxes on the page each time a particular situation occurred and was then able to see that his discomfort was related to his lifestyle. This enabled him to comply well with a programme to help relieve the problems that were leading to his poor quality of life and allowed him to participate in new and satisfying activities.

An example of this style of chart is shown in Appendix 12.2.

Communication charts

Communication charts can provide patients with a means to demonstrate their needs, whether these are physical, emotional or spiritual, and can help with the identification of what it is that will provide comfort and reassurance for them. General charts should be available for patients who are admitted to the ward at times when there are no staff available to assess their communication needs and deal with them, such as in the evening or at the weekend, or when waiting for the speech therapist to assess the situation. These may contain pages related to pain and other discomfort, feelings, activities of daily living, food and drinks, comfort needs, such as lighting, cushions, seating, spectacles, hearing aid, etc., and leisure activities – TV, music, reading materials, etc. They can take a variety of forms – picture only, words and pictures or words only, or there can be several sections to each page, or only one, depending on the patient's abilities, e.g. is there a visual defect; is there any cognitive impairment? It may be useful to include a page with the alphabet, and others with numbers, dates, etc.

It is important not to overwhelm the patient with too much information and, also, having a large book will discourage carers from using the charts. It is also helpful to include a page or two of guidelines for use, as people often imagine that patients will be searching through the book to find what they want to say when in fact, it is the carer who needs to be the facilitator, and ask the appropriate questions, directing the conversation. The charts may need to be created in English and another language, to make communication possible when there is no interpreter available. Preparing these charts with someone from that particular ethnic group will mean that the charts produced are culturally acceptable and do not contain anything that might be considered inappropriate. The helper can be a cultural worker or family member, who can also advise on individual issues that need to be included. For example, certain foodstuffs may need to be omitted or references to religious rites and rituals included.

A very useful computer program for developing communication charts is 'Boardmaker' (Mayer-Johnston, Inc., California: www.mayer-johnson.com). This affords the opportunity to show pictures and words, or either pictures or words alone, and translations are also available on the program for a wide variety of languages. It is important that people are able to convey their emotions and this program offers the opportunity to do this. Examples of two of the illustrations available are shown in Appendix 12.3. A personalised communication chart can be compiled using this software, ensuring that only material relevant to the individual patient's needs is included. This avoids the need for patients to expend a lot of energy, and makes compliance much more likely.

Communication charts should be personalised at the earliest opportunity, paying particular attention to why they are needed – to identify emotional issues; or for a particular procedure, such as monitoring blood transfusion or other treatment; or to assist discussion about a particular event, where closed questions are not enough.

Some patients will need more than basic communication charts to be able to express themselves, and the speech and language therapist (SALT) will advise in this situation. It is important to have a referral system arranged, and to work closely with the SALT department, in order to optimise the services available as quickly as possible. Some people can lose the ability to communicate over a very short period, and this can be extremely distressing at a time where communication is vital.

Eye-pointing charts, for people who have no other mobility and no speech, will be a useful alternative and although communication will be very limited using this method, by using carefully directed questions, and patience and perseverance, patients can feel that they can still have some autonomy.

Diaries

Diaries, as discussed in Chapter 12, can be used to monitor symptoms and allow patients to connect with their inner selves. They may contain charts of the daily activity programme for the management of symptoms and refer to planning, pacing, and prioritising, relaxation or breathing exercises. They may include instructions such as how to get dressed/undressed.

Another use of diaries is as an aide-mémoire. Staff and relatives should be encouraged to help with completing these, writing in times of activity sessions, who is visiting and when. This helps patients to feel more in control of their situation, being able to anticipate what will be happening and helping with recall of the day's/week's events.

Diaries can also be used to reflect the person's unique character, and may be used as tools to promote conversation with new people. They are also useful for continuity – relaying information when patients move between different environments in the course of their illness, such as home, hospital, nursing home, hospice. These communication diaries are like a personal identity card, recording the information that people would like to share about themselves, with those who are caring for them. Favourite foods, places, activities, colours, flowers and pets can all be recorded, with photos of family and friends. Everything can be labelled and people named, to help with recall and assist with conversation. It is important to record dislikes as well, to avoid frustration. Information may be related to their usual routines – the time that they like to get up; how they like to eat and drink, whether they like their food liquidised, hot or cold; whether they drink with a particular type of cup or straw; what leisure activities they have enjoyed or disliked. These books are cameos of people's lives, and will contain facts about individuals to help professional carers get to know them better, and so respect their personhood and their dignity (Chochinov et al 2005).

Diaries often contain photographs of patients participating in a variety of activities, and sometimes photos of the finished item. Patients have photographs taken of themselves with visitors and include these in their diary, which will eventually provide a record of this particular time and is often treasured by the relatives as a snapshot of their loved one and a lasting memory of their lives.

> Julie's husband was frustrated that she was unable to share with him the things she had been doing at day hospice. Her verbal communication had deteriorated rapidly and she was too overwhelmed with fatigue to try to talk. The therapist developed a personal diary for Julie, writing down all of the things she had been involved in that day and taking photographs of Julie enjoying her art sessions. This simple diary soon developed into a journal as Julie and her husband added to the photos and stories, and when she died he visited the therapist to say how much he appreciated having what had become a memory album of their last few months together.

Relationships

When people use externalising strategies to deal with their symptoms (e.g. pain, distress) this may manifest itself in increasing anger with others, resulting in an increase in interpersonal stress and tension in a relationship. Their inability to express fears and anxieties to relatives (Lugton 2002) can cause conflict and unresolved feelings, as can changes to normal routine, roles and responsibilities, and worries about financial issues. Elements of the life story will give valuable clues towards building an understanding of family dynamics and highlight why patients may feel the need to explain past behaviours to significant people in their lives, rekindle and reinstate lost relationships and to make amends.

They can discuss regrets, and anticipate and grieve for the end of their lives. Some people wish to have just one day where their family will treat them as they did before the illness.

Hilda's family looked after her very well. She really appreciated all their care, but when asked what she would like for her birthday she replied 'I just want you to treat me like me – the way you did before I was ill.' They did, and she had a wonderful day.

This is a time where friends may find it too difficult to cope with the close proximity of death and withdraw, but new friendships can be made, and often the depth of these, over a relatively short space of time, can be surprising and yet amazingly exhilarating for the patient.

Frances, day hospice patient: 'Although I have only known Ann for a short time, and we only met because we both have cancer, we feel that we've known each other for years and years. It's a very intense thing. We get great strength from each other.'

Where there are difficulties discussing the impact of the illness on people's lives, these may be related to fear of sharing anxieties and upsetting each other, in an effort to protect each other from hurt (Smith 1990, Syren et al 2006). Where relationships have been strained for some time, distancing and avoidance are common tactics used in order to ignore the real issues, adding a further loss – of a relationship – to the list of other losses experienced, and leading to loneliness and despair (Brown & McKenna 1999, Kissane et al 2001, Lichter 1991). Some patients experience anticipatory mourning, where they grieve for lost opportunities and their lost future. This may manifest itself in their withdrawal from contact with others, precipitating a social death and turning their faces to the wall, refusing any interventions. For relatives and carers, the experience of anticipatory grief can be a positive process, where people use the time left to work through and hopefully find satisfactory solutions to outstanding issues that may otherwise cause problems later in the grieving process. There is time to say what needs to be said, and for reconciliation to be achieved (Byock 1996). However, the paradoxical situation in which loved ones find themselves, where they are trying to maintain a relationship, whilst at the same time gradually withdrawing, can be very stressful, making communication strained.

There are several ways that carers can be involved, helping them to feel useful and supportive. Asking relatives to bring photographs and to help with dates and names for memory albums or a communication diary is one, and involving carers in rehabilitation issues such as activities of daily living or diary keeping (Kennett et al 2004) or suggesting that they share relaxation sessions at home are others.

Children can be involved in creative activities with parents and grandparents, such as artwork or music therapy, or interactive play using multisensory equipment, such as fibreoptic lights. Sharing videos, books and games will also help to make the experience of visiting a pleasurable memory for the child.

People need to feel that something of themselves will remain after their death. If there is no longer a physical presence, how can the things that made them what they were endure?

Apart from leaving last gifts for loved ones, they can be reassured that images in the form of photos around the house, or gardens that they have created and tended, plants that they have grown, and family traits and looks, amongst a whole host of other things, will all act as reminders.

Making the connection with patients

'Competent and effective end of life care means not only skilled practice in the science and techniques of pain and symptom control but also the art of building and sustaining relationships, and in the use of the self as a primary diagnostic and therapeutic instrument' (Boston et al 2001).

Professionals may use distancing, power and controlled emotion to maintain their role. This will be counterproductive in the communication process, resulting in superficial and ineffective interaction. To enable patients to take some control of their circumstances, and ensure that the communication process is a facilitative one, understanding their situation is the key (Carter et al 2004).

Good communication will encompass counselling skills, including creating a trusting and empathic atmosphere, and the observance of non-verbal communication, as described in Chapter 7. Picking up signs and signals and hearing what people are really saying and meaning is the key to successful interactions between individuals, enhancing core skills and giving a more holistic view of the situation. Listening to their life stories helps establish patients' perspectives (Carter et al 2004), and acknowledging the issues that are important and precious to patients helps them feel valued as people and strengthens the connection between the patient, the family and the professional (Chochinov et al 2005). Hopes and dreams that patients had for the future, and how the disruption of these plans has impacted on their lifestyle will also be highlighted (Carter et al 2004). In this way, patients are given the opportunity to communicate their feelings (Lichter 1991), their ways of coping with things in the past, and their reasons for their behaviours. For example, a person with mobility difficulties who would normally deal with anxieties by being active and perhaps going for long walks will become frustrated and upset if this coping mechanism is no longer an option. By connecting with the patient and the patient's story, another way to address the situation can be suggested.

One method of assessment that should be considered is communication through the senses. This is particularly useful with children, and is referred to in Appendix 12.4.

For professionals, communicating with colleagues, sharing stories and discussing feelings and experiences with others, such as in supervision sessions, can be a cathartic experience for the people connected with the patient.

Group work

The importance of communication as a process in group work is discussed in Chapter 1. It helps people to develop connections with themselves and others, and highlights who they are, defining the essence of those individuals and their spirituality. Listening to others, and sharing conversations related to their illness and the fact that they are dying, is one of the positive reasons patients give for coming to day hospice.

Jessie, talking about her experience in a day hospice group: 'When you're talking in a group, you find you have common ideas about things. Even if you are a quiet person, you can listen to the conversation and you hear people talking about the things you are thinking about, but might feel too shy to say. It helps to bring you out of yourself.'

Discussion in the social context about mortality can be made easier by the use of humour, allowing patients to talk about death and dying through the use of innuendo and non-verbal expressions. In this way, people can acknowledge their situation, but at the same time, distance themselves from it (Langley-Evans & Payne 1997).

Marion, day hospice: 'We can have a good laugh here!'

It is important to communicate with the other people involved with a patient – the patient's relatives and members of the multidisciplinary team – to arrange suitable times for activities and interventions, planning ahead and informing the patient the previous week. This will lessen the chance of interruption, or patients being forced to make the choice between participation in the group and having a bath or their hair done.

Providing information

For people to feel in control of their situation, they need to be able to express their concerns, identify their needs and understand how they can help themselves. To support them in making decisions and achieving these goals, they require the relevant information and all of this must be taught in a manner fitting to their own personal needs. The health professional can use narrative to offer examples of how this intervention has helped others, and how it can be introduced into the individual's lifestyle, encouraging participation by describing positive outcomes.

Written information is useful, as patients may not be able to fully understand or retain the details, because of fatigue, learning disability, information overload, anxiety, etc., or they may want to think it over. Checking up at the next session if they have understood and have been able to introduce the new ideas into their lifestyles will underline the salient points once more. Some people like to collect their own portfolio of information, and to take things home to share with others. This is useful where carers also need to be educated about the management of a particular issue and may underline the fact that patients have been told to pace themselves and incorporate periods of relaxation into their day. Care must be taken to supply as much or as little information as individual patients might need. People with memory problems may need more information, as it might need to be more detailed, whilst for those with learning difficulties, brief, explicit notes may be adequate (Rahman 2000).

Activities to enhance communication

Using activity as a catalyst for communication between the professional and the patient has been discussed in previous chapters. During activities-of-daily-living (ADL) sessions such as washing or dressing practice, there will be opportunities for making connections. Creativity is a powerful medium for communication and is discussed at length in Chapter 8.

The imminence of death and people's experience of the process of dying will heighten the meaning of their particular choice of occupation. These activities may be unique to that point in time and concerned with the preparation for death. They may be related to a number of factors:

- The need to continue with discrete activities and to keep going as before, for as long as possible (Chochinov et al 2005) will also preserve a sense of who they are.

> April wanted to be Mum to her 6-year-old from her hospice bed. She loved playing games with Josie when she came to visit, but missed the ritual of bedtime stories. The therapist helped her to record these on tape so that the night-time ritual that they had enjoyed together could continue, and suggested keeping in touch by text messages.

- Displaying photographs of people when they were well will demonstrate how they used to look and the sort of activities they enjoyed, and is particularly useful where people feel embarrassed or upset by their present body image and how others perceive them. Collage work, depicting a variety of aspects of their lifestyle will emphasise their personhood and improve self-esteem.
- Using either the activity or the created item as a way to say something to another person.

> Val had not been able to work since her illness began. She missed her friends at work and felt that she wanted the opportunity to have the retirement party that she had always planned. With the help of her husband, she planned a party and made and sent out individual invitations to all of her friends and work colleagues, with special messages for them all, thanking them for their love and support.

People can also discuss with others what they have been doing in an activity session, and this provides an alternative topic of conversation from the one related to illness, or it may act as a catalyst in the communication process, initiating conversation about a number of hitherto undisclosed issues. These can range from wishing to express thanks for care and love, to other, deeper concerns, such as seeking or offering reconciliation or forgiveness, or offering words of comfort, and messages of hope for the future. This can be shared through gift making, cards, letters, emails and memory albums.

- Finding closure and saying goodbye (Bye 1998). Writing as a form of communication is often a very acceptable alternative to the spoken word. Text can be reread and redrafted to provide a lasting record of an event or feelings, and is a tangible reminder of the sender. By describing techniques and showing examples, and listening, guiding and offering reassurance at each stage, activities such as letter writing, card and gift making and preparation of orders of service will allow people to express themselves and their feelings to the people who matter most.

> James was a doctor who had made many friends through his work in Africa. He kept in touch mainly through Christmas cards, but this year it would be especially difficult as James had recently discovered that he was terminally ill and could not write his usual letters with their

uplifting messages. He wanted let his friends know what was happening and felt that personal letters were the only way. Attentional fatigue and poor manual dexterity meant this was difficult so, together with the therapist, James wrote a basic letter on the computer for his many contacts and adapted it for his closest friends.

- Dealing with unfinished business and ensuring that roles and responsibilities are handed over in a satisfactory way. For example, tutoring someone else in how to deal with particular matters that have been the responsibility of the patient, e.g. developing a spread sheet to help families deal with household affairs such as paying bills, or drawing up an order-of-service programme with the patient can facilitate a conversation with the family about the practicalities of death – funeral arrangements, what the patient wants to leave to whom, contacting estranged relatives. Being able to make decisions about these issues enhances feelings of control and mastery over their situation.
- Confirming their unique identity for themselves, including their roles and status, and their place in time. This may involve activities that promote self-expression, or are based around stories that explain and make sense of events from the past. For example, life review, collage work and other creative activities representing the essence of that person.
- Confirming their existence to others, ensuring that aspects of themselves will endure over time and participating in activities that will be left as legacies, such as gift making, creating memory albums and boxes, letters and cards.

Miriam's daughter would be 5 soon and she went shopping with the therapist for a pattern and material to make a party dress. Miriam had recently decorated the little girl's bedroom and wanted to make some special things for it. She stencilled a coat rack and a pencil box with butterflies – Cara loved them since their visit to the butterfly farm – and made a little rocking cradle for the child's favourite doll.

When suggesting which activities would best serve the individual's needs, it is important that they should be given some time to consider these (Rahman 2000) and make their choices as to what their priorities are. Who do they most want to make a gift for or send a card to?

Memory making

'Death is a mirror that reflects one's life . . .' (de Hennezel 1997)

When people are reaching the end of their lives, they look back in order to search for what has made it all worthwhile. This process of appraisal at the end of life is considered a positive and meaningful exercise (Lichter 1993), allowing patients to communicate with their inner selves as they review their existence, and to communicate with others, both during the process and afterwards, in memories left as a legacy. These are stories that dying patients need to tell, and to pass on down the generations, keeping their memory alive. They can be presented as a scrapbook or memory box, but memory making can also develop from other activities, such as life-story work and reminiscence, diary keeping or creative art sessions. The perpetuation of links in the form of memories of loved ones who have died is considered a useful means of working through grief (Smith 2005) and tangible memories in the form of gifts and journals will be a lasting memorial that can be touched and cherished.

Sharing memories with others can recreate a mood, in the reader, of a certain time and place. The senses are stirred and emotions aroused, perhaps with the use of a familiar phrase, a photograph, a scent or an object that represents a connection with something shared and meaningful. They offer solace in the knowledge that they confirm a person's existence and provide material evidence of that life; they are enduring testaments to the roles that people had and the impact they made on the world and those around them (Byock 2002). Patients may be surprised at how stimulating sharing reminiscences with another person can be.

> Cathy talking about her reaction to the suggestion that she create a life-story book: 'When it was first suggested I thought I couldn't do it as I've never done anything like it before. My husband encouraged me to get on with the story and it encouraged us to talk about it and reminisce. I'm really pleased with it. It gave me a lot of satisfaction.'

For some people, relating the stories of the past is a liberating experience, allowing them the opportunity to assuage their guilt or regrets surrounding a particular event by building bridges and resolving past problems. Relationships can be strengthened by the sharing of treasured memories, enhancing emotional well-being and a sense of belonging and of being loved (Brady et al 1999). Anecdotes, which would be lost to future generations, can be recorded, including the person's involvement in certain historical events, or impressions of what it was like to live through a particular time such as the war, or man landing on the moon.

The influence they have had on others during their working lives – people that they have trained, mentored and guided, and their innovations – is of paramount importance for some, and needs to be shared and acknowledged. This can be a particularly useful approach with people who have no family and feel they are leaving no legacy (Pickrel 1989).

People want to be remembered in a positive way in order to bestow value and meaning on their existence, and that they have accomplished some, if not all, of their dreams and their goals. Personal achievements need to be shared and situations and behaviours explained, leading to resolution, spiritual fulfilment and peace.

By helping in the preparation of these legacies and sorting photographs or providing missing dates and details, relatives can assume a useful role at a time when they often feel deskilled and ineffective. Hearing or reading these recollections will nurture a deeper understanding of the people and their lives and so create the opportunity for a more empathic relationship between individuals.

Memory albums are created to encourage continuity, to record family history for future generations to enjoy. They confirm identities and give their creators a sense of control over the stories they tell and how they are told. For surviving relatives, they can serve as an aide-mémoire, providing something that those left behind can touch and caress, continuing their ties with their loved one as they work through their grief, by holding on to memories and emotions (Smith 2005) and perhaps stimulating the reframing of cherished connections in the future. They may be for the patient's children, whether they are adults, young people or babies, or even for children not yet born. This sharing of family anecdotes, about the children themselves, their place in the family structure, and the parts they played in significant occasions, will further establish their connections within their family, including cultural aspects and family rituals, cementing ties and enhancing their identity by defining their sense of who they are.

As with other forms of narrative, the development of a memory album is a dynamic process, often starting with musings and daydreaming about the past. Externalising these intimate stories requires assurances of confidentiality, supported by an established therapeutic relationship where supportive listening and good interpersonal skills will nurture an atmosphere of trust and help the teller to feel at ease. Voice tone and appropriate responses that offer reassurance will encourage continued participation, whilst sensitivity to emotional, psychological and spiritual issues that influence these stories will allow the dialogue to be directed by the listener.

Patients may have limited time in which they can participate in the production of their memory album. This may be because the end of their life is very near, or that they have limited resources or periods when they are fully conscious and aware. A flexible approach is very important here, as the patient will want to engage at every available opportunity and will expect this to be reciprocated (de Hennezel 1997).

Another way to make best use of time could be to leave 'homework' that patients can work on, say at night, with the help of other staff, or with relatives. Many patients who are very poorly will request that they be roused in order to work on their project, and seem able to find the energy to continue with this activity long after they lose their independence for other things. Patients need to be offered maximum practical support at this time, but must always feel that the project is still theirs. Underlining the fact that they are the ones making the choices, and that the helper is just the 'hands', is an acceptable compromise for patients.

Observation of non-verbal communication, such as body language and facial expression, will be useful in understanding the real emphasis of the story, and will reflect changes in energy levels and concentration. It can also be a useful indication of any discomfort, both physically and emotionally, allowing the listener to move towards winding up the session on a positive note, leaving the patient with a feeling of accomplishment. This is important, as negative feelings such as doubt, shame, guilt, fear or regret may be uncovered and expressed during the process and can lead to psychological distress and despondency if not addressed appropriately. People may feel that their life has been unremarkable, but by listening to their stories positive aspects of their lives can be identified and developed.

Facilitators must be aware that disclosure of negative issues may occur, often unexpectedly, and be aware of their personal and professional limitations, and when and where to seek assistance for the patient and for themselves. Emotional involvement can be difficult for professionals, particularly if they identify with particular issues in the patient's story and feel that it in some way mirrors an area in their own lives, or reflects a personal fear. The time that the whole process needs can also cause internal conflict for professionals, as planning and prioritising of this activity in relation to the needs of other patients or other aspects of their role, demand attention. Energy levels required, from both the physical and emotional perspectives for both patient and professional, also require careful consideration.

Reflections may relate to any period in people's lives. They may be connected to a very specific time, such as their childhood or working life, or to their child's life, or they may tell the story of the last few weeks of their illness and how important relationships were to them at that time. Some people may begin with a small cameo of a time in their life and progress to sharing stories of other times, which may or may not be connected. Others will have a very definite idea of the times they want to share, such as recording memories of their relationship with a child, often wanting to cover the whole of that child's life.

Process

The process for developing a memory album will be different for each person. It is important, however, to illustrate any suggestions about this activity with prepared examples that will demonstrate the wide choice of methods that can be used, and to identify how patients would like their memories to be recorded. These will also confirm that memory albums can be just a few pages long, but still tell the important stories. At this stage, people often want to take some time to consider the proposal and may want to discuss it with relatives and friends.

As well as showing examples, it is also useful to make suggestions about where to start, and to describe briefly how the album could develop, offering a few alternatives and emphasising that help will be given with choices related to the practical aspects, if required. For example, people may worry that they have no personal photographs to illustrate their book. This can be overcome by using material downloaded from the internet, or computer packages for clip art, or newspaper headlines from the past, or by accessing details from local reminiscence groups or library archives. If the stories are describing the experience of the illness, photographs can be taken of activities that the patient participates in at the hospice, such as creative activities or music therapy sessions, outings and theme days, and these can be added to the album.

Photographs are very useful prompts for starting this activity, after which the patients can take the lead, moving backwards and forwards through their stories and sometimes changing their remembered experiences in the process. At each stage, storytellers should be offered the typed transcripts for comment and correction, and perhaps the ideas for the next stage left with them to mull over.

They may choose several other ways to illustrate their stories and develop the mood that they want to convey. The words of significant songs or poems can be inserted, or favourite quotations from novels or films. Creative activities such as drawings, clip art, stickers, fabrics and a variety of papers, including handmade paper could be used to embellish the pages. Showing the transcripts in different styles of type and spacing will allow patients to chose the style that they feel suits their story best.

During the process, consideration can be given to the presentation of the finished album – how will it be contained? A ready-made photograph album could be used, or a journal sold for use as a scrap book. A variety of folders can also be used, and the style of cover (fabric, illustrated, paper and card), the colour and thickness of the pages, the size of the pages, how the photographs are mounted and displayed, how the sections are presented (chronologically, in order of importance) and what is to be shown on the opening page, can all be discussed either as the project is progressing, or at the end, whichever is the most appropriate. If the memory album is to be large, it will be best to work on sections at a time, varying between dictation and illustration in relation to energy and concentration levels.

Envelopes which hold wishes for the future can be pasted into the album, and extra pages can always be inserted at the back so that people feel that there is still scope to add to the book if they wish.

Creating memories is not necessarily a visual activity. Thoughts and reminiscences can be recorded on audiotape, or text messages can be sent. Music therapy sessions or bedtime stories for children can be taped, perhaps for a child unable to read yet. One particular patient was able to record commands on her chat box before she lost her speech, and her husband requested an audiotape of this after her death, reporting later that it had given him great comfort to remember his wife in this way.

Memories need not be represented by written or spoken words. Smell is a very powerful memory stimulant, and the scent of soap, perfume, herbs or cleaning materials, for example, can bring long-forgotten moods, emotions and memories flooding back. Likewise, touch can stimulate memory – the feel of velvet or a piece of someone special's clothes or maybe a baby blanket. Certain sounds – pieces of music for instance – or photographs or pictures or the taste of something from the past can all recreate experiences from another time. These items can be stored in boxes, allowing communication with the past through the senses. The container can be simple –

shoeboxes, small wooden or papier mâché chests and boxes – or larger and more elaborate versions available commercially from sources such as Barnardo's.

As time goes on, reaching for those memories can become more difficult, but the legacy of personal items such as jewellery, scarves, photographs and audiotapes will all help maintain a continued relationship with earlier times. The contents will be a reflection of someone's individuality – a representation of that person's essence of being, and the things that the person wanted to share and be remembered by. Children will want to have evidence of relationships, and memory boxes and albums will help consolidate their identity. Examples of what the contents might be are: when they started walking and talking, what they said and what happened, details of their birth – baby wrist band, their weight, hair colour, etc. – small items of clothing that they wore, favourite toys, and perhaps photographs of them playing with these toys or wearing these clothes.

Preparing these memories is a very emotionally charged experience. Patients will once again have to be assured of the confidentiality surrounding this type of activity, and offered privacy and support during the process. Once patients feel that the memory album is completed, arrangements are made with them regarding the safe storage of their work, and whether they want to give it to someone now, or if there is someone they have in mind to receive it after their death.

References

Abiven M 1995 The crisis of dying. European Journal of Palliative Care 2(1):29–32

Boston P, Towers A, Barnard D 2001 Embracing vulnerability: risk and empathy in palliative care. Journal of Palliative Care 17(4):248–253

Brady M J, Peterman A H, Fitchett G et al 1999 A case for including spirituality in quality of life measurement in oncology. Psycho-oncology 8:417–428

Brown R, McKenna H P 1999 Conceptual analysis of loneliness in dying patients. International Journal of Palliative Nursing 5(2):90–97

Bye R 1998 When clients are dying: occupational therapists' perspectives. Occupational Therapy Journal of Research 18(1):3–24

Byock I 1996 Beyond symptom management. European Journal of Palliative Medicine 3(3):125–130

Byock I 2002 The meaning and value of death. Journal of Palliative Medicine 5(2):279–288

Carter H, Macleod R, Brander P et al 2004 Living with a terminal illness: patients' priorities. Journal of Advanced Nursing 45(6):611–620

Chochinov H, Hack T, Hassard T et al 2005 Dignity therapy: a novel psychotherapeutic intervention for patients near the end of life. Journal of Clinical Oncology 23(24):5520–5525

Clinical Standards Board for Scotland (CSBS) 2002 Specialist palliative care. Standard 6. CSBS, Edinburgh

de Hennezel M 1997 Intimate death: how the dying teach us to live. Warner, London, p 100

Ellenberg E 2004 The recognition and respect of patient needs at the end of life. European Journal of Palliative Care 11(6):242–245

Head B 2005 Terminal restlessness as perceived by hospice professionals. American Journal of Hospice and Palliative Care 22(4):277–282

Kennett C, Harmer L, Tasker M 2004 Bringing the arts to the bedside. European Journal of Palliative Care 11(6):254–256

Kissane D W, Clarke D M, Street A F 2001 Demoralization syndrome – a relevant psychiatric diagnosis for palliative care. Journal of Palliative Care 17(1):12–21

Langley-Evans A, Payne S 1997 Light-hearted death talk in a palliative day care context. Journal of Advanced Nursing 26:1091–1097

Lichter I 1991 Some psychological causes of distress in the terminally ill. Palliative Medicine 5:138–146

Lichter I, Mooney J, Boyd M 1993 Biography as therapy. Palliative Medicine 7:133–137

Lugton J 2002 Communicating with dying people and their relatives. Radcliffe Medical Press, Oxford

Pickrel J 1989 'Tell me your story': using life review in counselling the terminally ill. Death Studies 13:127–135

Rahman H 2000 Journey of providing care in hospice: perspectives of occupational therapists. Qualitative Health Research 10(6):806–818

159

Smith N 1990 The impact of terminal illness on the family. Palliative Medicine 4:127–135

Smith S H 2005 Anticipatory grief and psychological adjustment to grieving in middle-aged children. American Journal of Hospice and Palliative Medicine 22(4):283–286

Syren S M, Saveman B I, Benzein E G 2006 Being a family in the midst of living and dying. Journal of Palliative Care 22(1):26–32

Appendix 12.1
Diary page

Kathryn Boog

Day	Date	
Activities		**Comments**
MORNING		
AFTERNOON		
EVENING		

Appendix 12.2
Illustrated diary page

Kathryn Boog

Monday 2nd June, 2003			
	Morning	Afternoon	Evening
☕			
🍽			
🍰			
🍲			
🍺			
☕💊			
😣			
😵			
😰			
😟			
😩			
🤸			

Appendix 12.3
Illustrations for a communication chart

Kathryn Boog

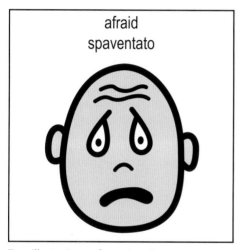

afraid
spaventato

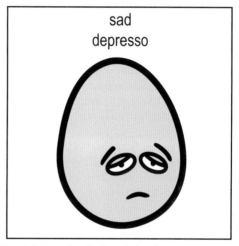

sad
depresso

Two illustrations of emotional expressions, available with 'Boardmaker' and showing translations.
(Picture Communication Symbols © 1981–2007 by Mayer-Johnson LLC. All Rights Reserved Worldwide. Used with permission.)

Appendix 12.4
Therapeutic communication with children

Claire Tester

Communication is never one way; it is understood and felt by another. Good communication skills contribute to a positive experience for the patient, family and staff (DoH 2004), whilst poor skills lead to dissatisfaction and unnecessary distress (DIPEx 2006, DoH 2003, Shiozaki et al 2005). This requires staff to be competent in effective communication (Egan 2002) and this has been highlighted as a training need especially in adult palliative care (Nyatanga 2001, NICE 2004). Although the main aim is to relieve the emotional, physical and spiritual suffering of the patient (Tan et al 2005), discussing death with a person can provoke anxiety in staff (Kubler Ross 1970), which in turn can lead to stress and burnout (Fallowfield et al 2002) when there is insufficient training. Cited difficulties of staff include the discussing and probing of patients' problems (Booth et al 1999), distress and embarrassment about what to say (Kubler Ross 1970), and a wish to protect the patient from distress (Fallowfield et al 2002). Such difficulties can cause conflict for staff (Barnes 2001) in withholding information. According to cultural and ethnic sensitivities, some relatives may encourage this behaviour (Shiozaki et al 2005). The avoidance of sensitive issues may create a sense of loneliness and isolation for the terminally ill person (Bluebond-Langner 1996, Chibnall et al 2002, Egan 2002).

When the patients are children or young people, the additional wish to protect them from further distress, and colluding with parents and staff in thinking that children or young people do not know what is happening to them, reinforce all of the above difficulties.

> Palliative care nurse: 'Although I work in an adult hospice, I know I couldn't work in a children's hospice because it would be too upsetting. I wouldn't know what to say.'

This raises another aspect – the fear of saying the wrong thing (Egan 2002, Kubler Ross 1970, Wilkinson & Roberts 2004). Communicating with children and young adults requires more than talking; it is necessary to listen to what is being said, as well as not being said, even when it is painful. It takes a sensitive listener who is prepared to listen, sit with pain, and enable children to unravel their thoughts and feelings. This is not easy and needs a serious intent to be aware of the child, and of oneself. There is no right or wrong way to communicate with a child but it does require an awareness of one's own communication skills. For example, if a child is providing a cue which the staff member finds difficult, the adult will block it. The child or young person understands this and develops thinking that the subject or question cannot be discussed, or at least not with this member of staff. Children and young people are sensitive to the way in which they are regarded and treated, and quickly discern who they feel comfortable with in discussing and sharing information, and who will respect their own feelings and questions. To begin a sincere communication about difficult emotional issues is also to recognise that you cannot always make things better, or provide resolutions. It also means that, being compassionate and sensitive, you will be affected by the emotional pain of the child.

There are different components or elements to communication to be aware of, which are listed here and intended as a guide. They are not limited to communicating with children, although the term 'child' will be used throughout. Neither are they limited to children who have verbal communication skills, but are appropriate for everyone. Indeed, children who are blind can be aware whether a person is focused upon them or not. Even if children are unable to initiate movement or to speak, the sensitivity of the staff working with them is communicated through these elements.

Elements of communication

These can be broadly banded into verbal communication relating to language, tone, pace, etc., and non-verbal communication relating to body language and signals (Wilkinson & Roberts 2004). Non-verbal communication may indicate something different from what is being said (Egan 2002).

Non-verbal communication
Distance
This is how close you sit to the child and relates to a comfortable personal space. This is approximately between 18 inches and 4 feet for an adult. With young children, there is a preference to sit alongside or near to them, without appearing intimidating. Desks and tables should be avoided unless the child chooses to sit behind a table.

Eye contact
Children often find it easier to talk if they are not looking directly at you, but when they look up they expect eye contact, which shows the adult is interested, focused and listening. This should not be staring at each other as it can feel threatening. It is important to be sensitive to cultural differences (Nyatanga 2001) which may view direct eye contact as unhelpful. Sitting at the same level is best, not standing over the child, so you are not appearing to look down or be superior (Wilkinson & Roberts 2004). This can mean sitting on the floor if the child is on the floor, but not sitting below the child.

Posture
This can convey your own emotional state, and that of the child. For example, drooped shoulders, with head lowered, can appear weary, and it is difficult for a child to talk to an adult who appears like this, as the adult already seems burdened. Equally, tension can be held in the body conveying emotional tension. Instead, your physical position should convey an attentive presence (Egan 2002) and readiness to listen, avoiding fidgeting.

Touch
Touch can be powerful (Wilkinson & Roberts 2004) but needs to be appropriate and acceptable. This is difficult to gauge with children, especially small children who might need a hug when upset. It is best to ask them: 'Would you like a hug?' There is a sensitivity to avoiding touch that might be misinterpreted by others. This is more difficult if a child initiates touch towards you. Again this should be carefully gauged and if inappropriate should be carefully redirected.

Gesture
Movements made can convey emotion and mood. These may include hand movements as well as facial movements such as smiling, or grimacing, etc. Anxiety might be shown in agitated movements, emotion spilling out into unconscious behaviour.

Verbal communication

This includes the language, the choice of words, and also the manner in which words are spoken (Wilkinson & Roberts 2004).

Language

This can vary depending upon cultural differences (Nyatanga 2001) and level of understanding. It is important to understand what is being said or implied and you may need to ask for an explanation, e.g. 'What does "stupid stuff" mean?'

Voice

The use of the voice includes tone, pitch, volume and speed in speaking, which convey emotion and affect the pace of the encounter. For example, a child was talking very quickly in an excited manner which was reflected back to him in a slower and gentle way: 'It sounds exciting'. Unfortunately, adults often patronise children, which creates a distance and resentment. Adults may vary their voice to match the content of the discussion and the mood of the child, but they should not be false.

Communication through play

Play is a means of expression and communication for young children. Cues in communication, both verbal and non-verbal, may also be expressed through spontaneous play. The practice of listening to a child, who may move quickly through different topics, requiring acute sensitivity in listening and identifying what is being said (Lanyado & Horne 1999), can be developed.

Facilitating communication

There are several techniques you might use to help in difficult encounters, including extremes of emotion, or resistance during a conversation. These include:

An agenda or model

In acknowledging that communication is a process (Egan 2002) there needs to be a beginning, a middle and an end (Lanyado & Horne 1999). This is held in your mind as an intention and encourages you to start, identify a middle, and then bring the process to a close that is helpful to the child. The end is not because you cannot bear to see the child upset and so you leave abruptly. A beginning is to encourage children to both tell their story and make sense of what is happening, e.g. 'Can you tell me how you got here?' Children may reply with an answer about transport, or about parents, or may explain their own understanding of the condition. This helps you to start from where the child is.

It is more helpful to follow the child's reply than to correct it with something like 'No, it was an ambulance.' What the child tells you, is what the child wishes you to know. If this is false, there will be a reason. This may emerge later. Accept what the child tells you, rather than imply an untruth.

Empathy

This is a way of feeling for the person, of compassion. Such acute sensitivity to another's emotion has the intention of not doing harm (Egan 2002) and can act as encouragement for more depth of discussion (Wilkinson & Roberts 2004). It enables a sharing of feeling, develops rapport and is respectful. This does not include pity, sympathy or your sadness, which are unhelpful to the child.

Listening

Listening requires an ability to hear what is conveyed verbally and non-verbally and to identify cues which can be explored (Egan 2002, Lanyado & Horne 1999, Wilkinson & Roberts 2004). It requires patience and an attention to what is being said so that it may be understood (Moylan 1994). Listening cannot be done properly if you are not focused on the child. Listening is different from hearing; it is thinking about what is being said and of the feelings and thoughts the child is conveying.

Pauses and silence
These are part of listening too, as understanding can be received in these spaces, acknowledging that in silence the non-verbal communication will still be going on (Egan 2002, Lanyado & Horne 1999). Such therapeutic space can encourage thinking or staying on one point made and can act as an encouragement for the child to continue, as you do not jump into the space attempting to fill it.

Encouragement
This shows active listening and interest, and can be conveyed by small sounds or words in acknowledgement of what is being said, or by actively encouraging the person to continue, e.g. 'right', 'yes' (Wilkinson & Roberts 2004).

Reflecting
This is repeating back what has just been said. It can act as a way of encouraging the person to speak more and is an example of active listening (Lanyado & Horne 1999, Wilkinson & Roberts 2004). It should be used sparingly. If, for example, a child says 'I can't think', the reflecting is to repeat this back with a question in the voice, so that the child is encouraged to explain a little more.

Questioning
Different questions can provoke different responses, whether 'closed' requiring a monosyllabic reply, or 'open' encouraging discussion (Booth et al 1999, Egan 2002, Wilkinson & Roberts 2004). Questions should be carefully phrased, because if they are too challenging they can cause a child to clam shut. The way in which a question is framed can be intimidating, e.g. repeating 'Why?' Space needs to be given for the person to reply and it is important that you do not try to answer the question yourself.

Clarification
Clarification is used to make sure that what has been said is understood by the interviewer. It prevents confusion and enables a point to be explored: 'How do you mean, it will all be over? . . . I don't quite understand.' Avoid assumptions and filling in with your own view.

Summarising
This is similar to reflection but enables a summing up of points, or main concerns discussed, at a point in the discussion. It also shows that you are keen to check that you have understood so far, e.g. 'So it seems you are worried about X, . . . and not sure how X will be, . . . and what will happen when Y finds out. Is that right?' This provides the opportunity for the child to agree, or disagree, and may extend these points. The child can see that you are interested and have listened correctly. This allows you to ask the child what can be done about these things, a plan forming between the two of you which might involve sharing with others, if the child permits.

Other considerations

Blocking behaviour
There are ways of communicating which actively block and inhibit good communication (Wilkinson & Roberts 2004). These may be deliberately used by you if you feel out of your depth, or there is something you do not want to discuss, or they may be unconsciously used. These can include;

- expressing and imposing your own feelings and values, e.g. 'I don't like that at all.'
- not allowing children to express their own emotions and feelings freely, even if negative and distressing to the child, e.g. 'Never mind, stop talking about that now and we'll do something cheerful.'
- changing the focus from the child to yourself, e.g. 'I had such a late night last night, I'm really tired.'
- using humour inappropriately, e.g. 'All that crying makes you look like a puffy red cloud!'
- over-identification, which can include thinking of your own past experience or thinking of the child as one of your own children, nieces, etc. (Egan 2002, Wilkinson & Roberts 2004); this is not thinking of the child's own feelings and experience, which is different.

Time

Time should not be a constraint, as it conveys an impression that there is insufficient time to listen or discuss the child's concerns, yet there needs to be an end, a satisfactory closing which is when a plan is made. For example: 'So, from the things we have talked about [list them] let's think together about what would help . . .'. Approx. 45 minutes to an hour is long enough to cover a beginning, a middle and an end, enabling a meaningful discussion with the child. For an initial discussion, a getting-to-know session of 20 minutes to half an hour is often plenty. Do not force a child to discuss or talk to you; children need to know that they can talk to you, and will take the opportunity when they are ready. This does not necessarily mean discussion occurs in a quiet room; it may be in the middle of a busy area, or on a bus journey. Care and attention are needed if there are others about, for the child should not be encouraged to confide, or to be vulnerable, in a public place, because the child will not feel safe with you. If the conversation develops you can say, 'I would like to talk to you more, shall we go into the quiet room?' Or, 'I can see these things are important/worrying for you, and it's difficult on the bus isn't it? When we get back can we talk some more?'

Reflection

It is helpful to reflect back upon such a discussion with the child, even to make some notes of it, being careful to write it down as it occurred and factually, not to write it as your interpretation. This helps to clarify what was being said and what was going on. Later this can be read through to obtain a deeper understanding and to help focus thinking on the next step, whether action is to be undertaken, or further clarity. If there are things the child has said you feel should be shared, you can, for example, say to the child: 'You know, I think because you are worried about the food, I think it would be a good idea to tell the cook, and the nurses about this so we could do something about it. Would that be alright?'

With parents

Aspects of collusion, denial, shock, anger, anticipatory grief and mourning are encountered in communicating with parents, and in turn parents communicating with their children (Mannoni 1987). It can be difficult not to become actively involved when the parents wish to shield their child from the truth (Bluebond-Langner 1996) especially when the child is already asking staff. It would be helpful to identify what is happening in any communication situation and to be able to discuss this with parents. In addition, it would be helpful to have an overview of how parents are coping and managing emotionally (Kristjanson & Ashcroft 1994). An understanding of different cultural and spiritual beliefs contributes to understanding how death is perceived (Ralston 1991, Nyatanga 2001) by different families so that sensitivity in communicating can be developed further.

References

Barnes K 2001 Staff stress in the children's hospice: causes, effects and coping strategies. International Journal of Palliative Nursing 7(5):248–254

Bluebond-Langner M 1996 In the shadow of illness – parents and siblings of the chronically ill child. Princeton University Press, New Jersey

Booth K, Maguire P, Hillier V 1999 Measurement of communication skills in cancer care: myth or reality? Journal of Advanced Nursing 30(5):1073–1079

Chibnall J, Videen S, Duckro P et al 2002 Psychosocial–spiritual correlates of death distress in patients with life-threatening medical conditions. Palliative Medicine 16:331–338

Department of Health 2003 Independent Complaints Advocacy Service (ICAS). Online. Available: http://www.dh.gov.uk

Department of Health 2004 Patient and public involvement in health: the evidence for policy implementation. Online. Available: http://www.dh.gov.uk

DIPEx 2006 Patients' perspectives. Online. Available: http://www.dipex.com

Egan G 2002 The skilled helper. Brooks/Cole, California

Fallowfield L, Jenkins V, Beveridge H 2002 Truth may hurt but deceit hurts more: communication in palliative care. Palliative Medicine 16:297–303

Kristjanson L, Ashcroft T 1994 The family's cancer journey: a literature review. Cancer Nursing 17(1): 1–17

Kubler Ross E 1970 On death and dying. Routledge, London

Lanyado M, Horne A 1999 The handbook of child and adolescent psychotherapy. Routledge, London

Mannoni M 1987 The child, his 'illness' and the others. Karnac, London

Moylan D 1994 The dangers of contagion: projective identification processes in institutions. In: Obholzer A, Roberts V Z (eds) The unconscious at work: stress in the human services. Routledge, London, ch 5

NICE 2004 Supportive and palliative care service guidance manual. NHS, London

Nyatanga B 2001 Why is it so difficult to die? Mark Allen Publishing, London

Ralston P 1991 Reflections of being. North Atlantic Books, California

Shiozaki M, Morita T, Hirai K et al 2005 Why are bereaved family members dissatisfied with specialized inpatient palliative care service? A nationwide qualitative study. Palliative Medicine 19:319–327

Tan A, Zimmermann C, Rodin G 2005 Interpersonal processes in palliative care: an attachment perspective on the patient–clinician relationship. Palliative Medicine 19(2):143–150

Wilkinson S, Roberts E 2004 Communication skills course. (CD-Rom) Marie Curie Cancer Care, London

Section 3

How to survive as staff

Hearts and minds – how the unconscious affects us

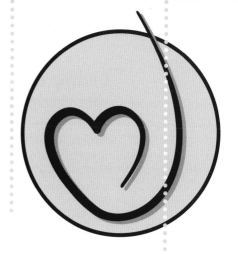

Claire Tester

They all said 'Hallo', and felt awkward and unhappy suddenly, because it was a sort of good-bye they were saying, and they didn't want to think about it.

A A Milne, *The House at Pooh Corner*

Key words

conscious; unconscious; thoughts; feelings; behaviour; emotions; splitting; projection; introjection

Chapter contents

13

Death is usually only considered when someone close to us dies. This usually does not happen very often, but it does happen to us all. When it does we are thrown into an emotional crisis of grief and mourning and need time to adjust to the impact of death and loss. The closer we are to the person who has died the more significant the impact. The impact is upon our own emotional life, our own feelings, and is stored as emotional experiences. Such experiences contribute to one's being, along with all of the other experiences in life reaching back into childhood. Memories are stored with emotional feeling and thinking both conscious and unconscious. Unwittingly we carry these memory banks around, unable to leave them behind.

How does this affect health professionals who are working in palliative care, working with children or adults who have a life-limiting condition, or are terminally ill? Do any of them really keep personal experiences, feelings and emotions out of their work and vice versa? Some of the difficulties of working in this environment will be considered with regard to the effect upon the unconscious and conscious thoughts and feelings. It is not the intention to seek pathology in oneself or one's colleagues, but to become consciously aware of how behaviour is unconsciously affected.

Living with dying

In palliative care, the health professional is surrounded by individuals who all have a life-limiting condition. When someone reaches the terminal stage the person's life may be measured in days or hours. Relatives are often distressed and already grieving. Emotions can run high, although there is often a calm and a quiet efficiency which health professionals employ. This is distressing and emotionally draining for staff, whether it is felt at the time or later in the evening or the next day. In fact when working with dying people and their loved ones, balancing care with respecting the need for privacy, the staff member will appear confident, attentive and compassionate. Such sensitivity comes with a price; that is, the emotional cost and toll which accrues over time upon the member of staff. Working in palliative care demands more than practical expertise; the human qualities of caring, consideration and compassion are needed. As relationships are formed in caring for people and getting to know them, their deterioration and death is felt keenly by staff.

> A child had died and the mother had requested a particular staff member, Anne, to help bathe and wash her child. The mother was unwilling to involve any other staff initially. Afterwards Anne was making tea to take to the mother, and was asked by a colleague if she had a cold. 'No. I am crying,' she said to the surprised colleague. 'But I thought you were doing so well,' came the reply. 'I am,' said Anne, 'but it's difficult, and I don't feel I can cry in front of the mum.'

Health professionals are meant to maintain a professional approach at all times and this has come to imply that emotions are not to be shown to patients or their families. This can also include colleagues and managers. It can be perceived as a sign of weakness by some staff. 'I think it's a sign of not coping. If you get upset you shouldn't be in the job,' was the opinion of one staff nurse in palliative care. Is this true, that to be effective and work in palliative care feelings should be kept under control and hidden? Menzies (1960) observed nurses working with very ill adults. The nurses' strong feelings and anxieties were controlled by institutional defences such as cleaning, keeping busy and keeping order.

There is a need for recognition that staff are affected by grief too, that they have feelings, and are affected. However, this is not universally considered. Staff may become demoralised, may feel deskilled and useless, and can feel isolated amongst their colleagues. How and why does this happen at all in palliative care, when the accent on the approach is to be considerate, and thoughtful of another's needs? It has been remarked that to have such a chapter in this book, on thinking of how staff are affected is 'self-indulgent'. Arguably this is in fact to be wisely selfish (Dalai Lama 2004), for the way in which staff feel directly affects their work.

Example

A situation occurred for the author which caused her to reflect and to try and understand her behaviour on that day. This is described in the first person.

A colleague and I were due to hold a training day in moving and handling for staff, at a children's hospice. This was the first time that the two of us would be working together as trainers for the whole day, although we knew each other and had a good working relationship. We had had little time to plan for the training day and there were still aspects of the day that we needed to prepare: organising chairs, preparing information packs, setting up the overhead projector, cueing up video clips, etc. The course was due to start at 9 a.m. and we had agreed that we would meet at our usual start time of 7.30 a.m.

The hospice is usually a busy place, even in the morning as staff arrive, the night staff hand over to them, and the domestic staff have already begun their work. Families are usually up and breakfasting or seeing their children, and of course the bedrooms have children in them. There are lights and different sounds, but on this morning, staff were all coming in for 9 a.m. for a training day, and no children or families were staying. There was only one nurse on duty for emergency cover. All this I knew as I entered through the back door of the hospice, which was dark and silent. So I was surprised to encounter a father standing in the corridor, just outside one of the bathrooms where the lights were on. He was talking to the chaplain, who I was also surprised to see. As I put my bag down in the office after saying 'Hallo' to both of them, the chaplain came to tell me that a child had died that morning at home and been brought into the hospice. The nurse on duty had telephoned the chaplain, before setting off herself to accompany the family to the hospice. I immediately went to give my condolences to the father, still standing in the corridor. He was looking towards the bathroom. The door was open and I saw the mother and the 2-year-old child who had just died. The nurse was there removing dressings on the child who was being undressed for a bath, which was running. I went in as the mother and nurse acknowledged me. I gave the mother an embrace and looked at her little boy, who appeared so vulnerable. Realising that the child needed to be bathed and too that there were no other staff to assist, I offered my help. The mother explained that she and the father wanted this quiet time alone with their son to bathe and dress him. The nurse and I withdrew. I was relieved that I was not needed as I still had so much to do for the training course, and I thought 'Right I must get on,' so I set off to begin the moving of furniture etc. in the room upstairs. I carried on, expecting my colleague to appear at any time but she did not. In fact, it was when everything was done and I went downstairs to make coffee that I saw her sitting talking to another member of staff. She still had her coat on.

My colleagues have told me that I am an easy person to get on with, and I have good relationships with them all. But I could feel myself becoming indignant and difficult, as I asked her where she had been. She explained that she had been held up in traffic and had been met at the door by the chaplain who had broken the news of the death of the child to her. She said that she thought I was talking to the nurse, and that she was not aware I had been setting up for the day's training. I asked for her help saying firmly that it didn't seem fair that I had been getting everything together on my own. She then in turn became indignant and this tone regrettably was set between us for the whole day. The attendees on the course were also aware of it. It was not until I began to reflect upon why my relationship with my colleague had been so different on that day that I came to realise what had happened unconsciously that morning.

Reflection

I had not been prepared in any way for encountering the child who had died and his parents that morning. I had literally walked unawares into the situation. This meant I encountered this lovely child whom I had known living, who had died just 2 hours before. The grief of his parents was palpable and raw. I did not allow myself to process the shock. I found it hard to accept the situation but believed myself to have processed it. I was vaguely aware of my feeling that it did not seem right or fair that such a beautiful small child and his loving parents should have to suffer so much. It all seemed wrong. Nothing seemed right. It was not fair. After saying goodbye to the child and his parents downstairs I did not allow myself time to stop and think. I believed myself to be switching off and focusing on what had to be done; that is, preparing for the training day which would go ahead. In retrospect I can see that as I carried out the tasks my thinking of 'it's not fair' was projected towards my colleague who had left me to do these chores. The depth and strength of my unconscious feelings about the child became directed consciously towards my colleague. It was all her fault, and nothing seemed fair. When I saw her I projected my anger and indignant feelings of 'it's not fair' into her. I did not link such a strong feeling with the dead child and his family at all, only that of a feeling that my colleague had let me down. She took this in, as I got rid of this feeling, she carried it and became indignant. She said she felt that I was not being fair.

My colleague had been hurrying as she was delayed in her journey. But she was met by the chaplain. The bad news she received stopped her and quite rightly she was given time to talk to the chaplain about the child, and to come to terms with what had happened. She was able to discuss her feelings a little. When she encountered me, I must have appeared uncaring and impatient. I thought I was doing my job, and that I had accommodated events which had occurred. I thought I had it all under control, but the emotions I had pushed down into my unconscious were trying to get out, were being got rid off by me as I could not bear them. I became angry with my colleague, when really I was angry and still in shock about the little boy dying and of it all being wrong. I put the strength of these emotions into blame upon my colleague.

Understanding the process

Klein (1998) identified a splitting of the emotions at an unconscious level. Klein upheld that when something is unbearable, intolerable or difficult if not impossible to understand or accept, it cannot be borne. It has to be got rid of; it is repelled at an unconscious level; it is too much to take in, because it is painful. The painful part of the emotions is split off and the 'good' part kept whilst the 'bad' is got rid of. As early as 1911, Freud had identified that a person would unconsciously be drawn to pleasure rather than pain (Freud 1984). In getting rid of such negative emotions we project them out. But if they have been projected out, where do these negative emotions go? What happens to pain, resentment, anger, frustration, sorrow, and other negative emotions? They are projected into someone or something else. Projection can be done unwittingly by the person holding these feelings. Getting rid of strong unwanted feelings can be through anger, or even silently and felt by another. They can be felt by a whole room if the projection is strong enough. There is discomfort, or even rising anger felt by the recipient. It may also be depression or overwhelming sadness. If the recipient rejects the feelings, they are passed along again. This goes some way to explaining why and how someone will go home and become suddenly angry over a small thing with a partner, the children or a pet.

> Nurse: 'I always go out and give the dustbin a good kick at the end of a bad day. I just don't want to think about all the rotten things that have occurred. I keep them at a distance and then take it out on the dustbin.'

Sometimes one can become aware of feelings, of oneself or of another, as the door is slammed. But feelings can be projected silently and unconsciously so that there is no awareness of them. They can be projected into someone else. In this way the intolerable, unbearable feelings and emotions are located in someone else. They can be felt by the person and, as they are felt, they can be introjected and owned by them as their own feelings. The person who receives the projection may hold it in (introject) and project it out later, perhaps at home, or not tolerate it at all and project it out at the workplace. This can be batted about in a workplace setting and may reinforce existing dynamics in the workplace. Emotions, and strong feelings do go some-where. The harder they are to bear the more likely they are to be split off and projected out, into someone else. Thinking of the situation which occurred with a colleague, it was only after long reflection that the process of splitting, projection and introjection was recognised, and a sincere apology given.

Working in palliative care

In working with people who have a life-limiting condition, or may be at their terminal stage, health professionals are surrounded by what is unbearable and intolerable for most of us to consider, our own mortality and that of others. The primitive anxiety of survival is aroused, albeit unconsciously. Menzies (1960) observed that nurses tending to very ill patients all shared a similar behaviour: they attempted to keep an emotional distance from their patients, which was stressful.

As our motivational force is to survive (Bowlby 1997), to live, the threat of dying or its proximity creates anxiety and fear. This is encountered in families and patients. It can also be present in staff, although this is not obvious.

A young child with a life-limiting condition fell over and cut her lip. A new member of staff at the hospice was with the child, and picking her up quickly she ran to the staff room crying out that she needed help as the child was bleeding. An older experienced staff member went to assist. The child had her mouth wiped and all was well, but the member of staff was anxious and panicky, and needed some considerable time to calm and to be reassured that all was well. In discussion afterwards, she admitted that she was worried that the child might have died and that the appearance of blood had caused her to panic. This thought that the child might die was at the back of her mind at all times she said. She openly acknowledged that if the child had not had a life-limiting condition she would have reacted in a different way, calmer and without seeking assistance. It was the anxiety and underlying tension of being alert to a child dying in her presence, and in her care, which was triggered for this staff member.

Our defence mechanisms spring into action, denying our own anxiety and helping us to cope. Defences are unconscious, but as they keep anxiety at bay they can be resistant to change (Mosse 2002) and may be adopted as a form of organisational behaviour. Defence mechanisms can be helpful but not always to others around us, for they act as a form of denying that something is going on. Being active and busy can be a form of defensive behaviour. The busier the environment, and the bigger the environment, the more the sense of isolation felt when feelings are reflected upon. Difficult emotions get through unconsciously to individuals who are there. This can be anywhere, but working in palliative care it needs to be acknowledged that there are negative and difficult emotions in abundance.

Making the unconscious conscious

Freud identified the unconscious as being a 'hidden aspect of mental life' (Halton 2002) which influences conscious emotional and thinking processes. The term 'Freudian slip' is given to the idea of things said as if by accident revealing the true thought or feeling of the speaker. Dreams also are an aspect of the unconscious. Each of us has an unconscious which can also become part of a shared or collective unconscious when behaviours are shared, and systems created. Obholzer (2002) writes:

'In the unconscious there is no such concept as "health" . . . but there is the concept of "death" and in our constant attempt to keep this anxiety repressed, we use various unconscious defence mechanisms, including the creation of social systems to serve the defensive function. Indeed, our health service might be more accurately called a "keep-death-at-bay" service.'

'I hate hospitals. My grandfather went into one and when he came out he was dead.'
(Baldrick in *Blackadder Goes Forth*, **Richard Curtis & Ben Elton 1989**)

Some defences can be healthy and helpful. For example, a fire officer commented, 'We always have to have a laugh and make a joke of it before we return to the station. No matter how bad it's been we have to let off the pressure, even though it's black humour half the time. No one else would find it funny.' Other defences such as keeping busy can get in the way and over time be harmful to individual staff members.

A nurse had spent the morning with bereaved parents who had placed their baby in the coffin, and escorted the parents and the coffin to the hearse. As the hearse drove away, a senior member of staff asked the nurse to complete the file, and to tidy the room the infant had used. Other members of staff were all occupied and not available to help. At the end of the shift the nurse left in tears exclaiming that 'everyone was cold and heartless'.

How and when are defensive mechanisms, projections and introjections used? It is helpful to be aware of when these are being used, and to become conscious of one's own feelings, and the feelings of others. It is not the intention to seek pathology or problems in the workplace nor in individuals, but just to raise an awareness, a healthy awareness in order to encourage the maintenance of a healthy emotional state. For in denying the emotional build-up which can occur in the unconscious, feelings and emotions can be stored which can become damaging to the individual.

Some examples of defence behaviour

Busy, busy, busy!

Therapist: 'There was a funeral service held at a hospice for a child who had died. Parents of other children known to the hospice came dressed in black for this service. They were very tearful as they knew such a time would come for them and their own children. The parents and children not involved with the service were kept separate by staff in another part of the building with loud music and television, and games, or they went out. The bedrooms between the two ends of the building needed cleaning for the children arriving in the afternoon. There were two extreme ends of life that morning – the dead and mourning, and the living. As staff, we were in the middle. I remember feeling that I just wanted to be busy and take my mind of it all. I think we all did as we all helped with the cleaning, working really hard, with so much energy, and no one talking about the service. Afterwards one of the nurses said we all needed rewarding and made a big pot of coffee and bought chocolate, but it was comfort food really. By being really busy and active we got through that morning, and didn't have to think about it. In fact everyone was quite positive about what they were doing.'

Such 'busy-ness' can negate the feelings of others too. As one occupational therapist said, 'I went in to see Mr T. but he wasn't in his bed, all of his things had gone. I asked at the nurses' station and they said he had died in the night and was in the mortuary. I used to see that man every day, and they knew that but no one had thought to tell me. They had just tidied everything away as if he was never there.'

Smiling

Being cheerful, and loudly commenting on the weather can be a defence. Everything is pleasant and nothing awful is happening or going to happen. This includes smiling too. Speck (2002) described the 'chronic niceness' of staff in hospices. This 'niceness' denies the pain and difficulty of working with dying people, and of strong negative emotions. Such smiling and niceness act as a defence, not to let pain in nor to let it show. A smiling and cheerful face can act as a barrier with a patient as if the staff member is saying, 'Don't upset me.' It can be difficult to be nice and cheerful all of the time, so the negative feelings are 'split off' unconsciously in order to maintain the nice, smiling friendly approach throughout the organisation. This can be viewed as a form of organisational behaviour, and the splitting off of negative emotions can become an institutional dynamic, a sort of unwritten law that someone or something is deserving of the negative. This is commonly perceived as managers being at fault. Occasionally it might be individual staff members who introject and carry the negative emotions, being perceived as negative at work. This can lead to 'scapegoating', wherein an individual has accumulated so much negativity that the person is perceived as being the negative influence within a workplace and has to leave. Ironically this person may be able to voice uncomfortable truths which cannot be heard by others, but which identify defensive behaviour in the workplace. Depending on how well-defended the other workers are, this person may not be heard. This echoes the position of a 'whistle blower'.

Cleanliness

Cleanliness – the activity of keeping everything clean and tidy – is to reduce infection, but can be seen as a defensive behaviour of keeping sickness and mess at bay and out of sight. It involves staff in following infection controls and protocols in the normal run of the day as part of a systems control, but can extend to an administrator's order for new paintwork every 2 years, of increased cleaning staff, and of regularly changing furniture and fittings. 'Cleanliness is next to godliness,' commented a staff member when cleaning a room as the child lay on the bed.

> Therapist: 'Looking at the architect's plan for the hospice building, the sluice was next to the domestics' cleaning stores, which was next to the room used to place people when they have died before they are taken to a funeral parlour. On the other side of this room was a store. It was the end of the building for cleaning and tidying the mess, and keeping things out of sight.'

There are strong negative emotions running as an undercurrent when working with children and adults who are dying. There is a belief that can occur which is that no harm will come to staff working in this environment, as if working in a specific field provides an immune system to it.

> A young woman who had been an active fund-raiser for a spinal injuries unit suffered a spinal injury whilst on honeymoon, which left her paralysed. She said that she could not understand why this had happened when she had done so much for others with spinal injuries. 'It shouldn't have happened, not when I've done so much for the spinal injuries unit,' she said indignantly.

When a serious illness or death occurs amongst the families of staff, or to staff members themselves, the impact can be profound. As one member of staff remarked, 'It's so much harder when it happens to one of us, it's like there is no let-up from illness and dying at all. You can't keep it out then can you?'

Thinking back to the opening paragraph of this chapter, of the emotional impact when someone dies, staff working with people who have a life-limiting condition, or are terminally ill, are affected. However, this is not always recognised. In fact people who appear to cope, to take it all in their stride, are often perceived as being in control and professional. There is an argument that, if there is no acknowledgement by individuals of the stress they are under and unconsciously accumulating, their own health begins to suffer.

'Attempting to suppress or deny the personal impact can be stressful, leading to fatigue, sickness, compensatory over-activity, loss of effectiveness at work and at home – together with other symptoms often referred to as burnout' (Speck 2002). Another aspect is the trigger for one's own past experiences that can occur when working with people. This trigger can be a situation one has experienced, e.g. the death of one's mother in a hospice, or a condition similar to that of the similarly aged patient one is working with. It could also be a similarity, perhaps of character or even likeness, to a member of one's own family or friends. This is transference, and counter-transference when the other person's feelings are perceived as one's own. Patients and their families also unwittingly use transference and counter-transference with the staff. These triggers can act as a personal link with a patient which would not be there if it were not for one's own experiences. Any unresolved feelings and emotions which are triggered can rise to the surface and can be re-experienced. This is often a shock and outwith the person's control as feelings and emotions rise through the unconscious. 'We are not as solid as we think', remarked Ben Okri, poet, when his mother died. Staff may choose to work in palliative care because of their own personal experiences. In this way they may be unconsciously seeking to achieve some resolution of past difficulties (Main 1968).

Pain and emotion are perceived as a can of worms which, once opened, burrow into everything and everyone, or like Pandora's box, once opened the 'bad' flies out uncontrollably and unrestrained. This threatens the cheerfulness of staff, and the existing defences and controlling behaviour. This is the belief for keeping the lid on. When a visiting nurse to a hospice was briefed upon a terminally ill child she was about to work with, she commented, 'Oh it's alright, I've worked with a lot of dying children and children who have died. I'm used to it all now.' The point is that it is not alright, it is not normal and not usual. To become insensitive or immune to it is not healthy. Time and support with acknowledgement of the difficulties and pain inherent in the work need to be given to staff (Mawson 2002) with the acceptance and understanding by managers that it is not a sign of weakness.

Some considerations for support

- As an individual – to reflect, to think and recognise one's own feelings at a conscious level. It is very helpful to consider one's feelings and experiences at the end of the day, and if need be to discuss them with another colleague.
- One-to-one discussion with a colleague – to talk, share and acknowledge difficulties. This can be informally, or in a peer review, or supervision session.
- Case presentations and studies – these can be helpful in discussing all aspects of a case with a group of staff. This can include the impact the person and family are having on the staff. The way in which such a meeting is chaired is important in supporting staff in discussions.
- Team meetings – these are opportunities for sharing and communicating as different team members contribute. As there are different professions bringing different skills and views to the work of the team, it is important that the team members understand the roles of each member. As staff can change, this exercise needs to be repeated regularly.

- Staff support meetings – ideally these would be with a trained facilitator who is neutral and outside of the team. Such a meeting allows a supported discussion to take place in a 'safe' setting. These meetings are confidential.
- Counselling – to meet a counsellor is neither a sign of weakness nor of difficulty but a recognition by an individual that emotions can build up. A counsellor can help a person reflect and discuss aspects of work, and the impact of home and family life. In this way emotions introjected can be consciously identified rather than churned back into home or the workplace.
- Reflective diary/accounts – it can be very hard to find the time in a busy day to write a reflective account. This may not need to occur every day but is a helpful experience.

Nurse: 'In the summertime six children known to the ward died. Not all of them died at the hospital, some died at a hospice, and one died at home. The last child who died was a 9-month-old baby whom I had been working with. They had visited the unit once and did not meet many staff. The child died suddenly and it was unexpected. It was the parents' first child and they were devastated. I ended up spending a lot of time with them as so few staff knew them. I was so upset, and felt so overwhelmed. I had not processed my thinking and feelings at all. I did not realise how I was feeling until one day when I just burst into tears at work, and decided to write down what was happening. I just didn't want to go home to my kids like that. Actually I was ready to give up my job.'

Staff often feel deskilled and powerless in not being able to prevent the death of a patient. Such helplessness can be distressing. Obholzer (2002, p. 174) writes that 'staff are ill prepared for this (powerlessness) in their training . . . this then expresses itself as illness, absenteeism, high staff turnover, low morale, [and] poor time keeping'. Care needs to be taken not to personalise issues in the workplace that probably belong to the whole group. To repeat, it is not the intention of the author to seek pathology in the workplace. All staff need support – this includes managers, and students too. Students are usually on short placements and are expected to quickly adapt to an environment and to contribute within it whilst being assessed doing so. Students are also seen as not a part of the established staff group and their needs are not always viewed in the same light. This can be reinforced by the students themselves, who are wanting to appear as if coping and able to work under pressure, for assessment marks. The attitude and approach of the supervisor can make a difference in this regard.

Conclusion

Working in palliative care is stressful, although the stress and the anxiety may be well defended amongst the cheerfulness and smiling of the staff. The staff who deny the existence of such primitive anxieties about death, which are in the unconscious, are deluding themselves. They may be managers or staff. Seldom are they new staff with such an attitude. New staff are able to see more clearly the difficulties and to try their hardest to 'fit in and conform'. Some defences are useful, others less so. Support and awareness of one's feelings and emotions, and the ability to support others and to share experiences are helpful.

> A member of staff who had worked at a hospice for 8 years returned after a year for a service of remembering. She said to a former colleague, 'When you don't work in this place any more, you can see what goes on very clearly. It's hard, it really is upsetting. I don't know how I managed to work here. To think, I even enjoyed it.'

The next chapter considers how one finds meaning and purpose in working in palliative care.

References

Bowlby J 1997 Attachment and loss, 2nd edn. Pimlico, London, vol 1

Dalai Lama 1997 The way to freedom. Thorsons, London

Freud S 1984 On metapsychology: the theory of psychoanalysis. Beyond the pleasure principle, the ego and id, and other works. Translated by James Strachey (1955) Penguin, London

Halton W 2002 Some unconscious aspects of organizational life. In: Obholzer A, Zagier-Roberts V (eds) The unconscious at work. Brunner-Routledge, London

Klein M 1998 The psycho-analysis of children. Karnac, London

Main T 1968 The ailment. In: Barnes E (ed) Psychosocial nursing: studies from the Cassel hospital. Tavistock Publications, London

Mawson C 2002 Work with damaged children. In: Obholzer A, Zagier-Roberts V (eds) The unconscious at work. Brunner-Routledge, London

Menzies I E P 1960 The function of social systems as a defense against anxiety: an empirical study of the nursing service of a general hospital. In: Trist E, Murray H (eds) The social engagement of social science: Vol. 1 The socio-psychological perspective. Free Association, London

Milne A A 1995 The house at pooh corner. Methuen Children's Books, London, p 165

Mosse J 2002 The institutional roots of consulting to institutions. In: Obholzer A, Zagier-Roberts V (eds) The unconscious at work. Brunner-Routledge, London

Obholzer A 2002 Managing social anxieties in public sector organizations. In: Obholzer A, Zagier-Roberts V (eds) The unconscious at work. Brunner-Routledge, London, p 171

Speck P 2002 Working with dying people. In: Obholzer A, Zagier-Roberts V (eds) The unconscious at work. Brunner-Routledge, London, p 97

Keeping going – as staff

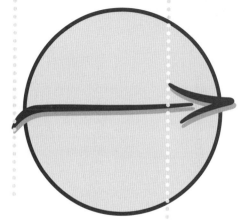

Claire Tester

Key words

emotional toll; deskilling; sensitivity; defensive behaviour; unconscious; grief; compassion fatigue; burnout; motivation

Chapter contents

Introduction

14

In acknowledging that there is pain, distress, sadness and grief in palliative care, why does anyone want to work in this field? In Chapter 13 on the role of the unconscious, it has been discussed that the motivational need to survive is paramount for us all, in any situation, and how difficult it can be to work with people who are terminally ill, or have life-limiting conditions. It can also be very rewarding work, and staff members are often very committed and hard working to provide the highest standard of care (Speck 2002, p. 97). This chapter will be looking at the personal emotional toll on staff, of how deskilling can occur, and recognising the signs and symptoms on the way to 'burnout'. Burnout and compassion fatigue will be explained. Strategies and positive ways of keeping going are provided in Appendix 14.1. Thinking about the impact upon staff as individuals, and of how all of them are different yet still in possession of their own sensitivities and feelings, rather than automata, is regrettably still a relatively new idea. What does it take to be a professional is still being debated in staff rooms. The idea of the 'stiff upper lip' is perpetuated by different staff disciplines and managers, whilst the absence of it can lead to the accusation of being 'emotionally over-involved' (Mawson 2002).

> Nurse: 'At one point I had two supervisors whose sessions overlapped because one was leaving. The first told me that I was too sensitive to work in palliative care, and the second told me that my sensitivity was an asset for working in palliative care.'

Menzies (1960) looked at staff turnover in nursing and observed that staff who were both sensitive and able to contribute positively to their patients were also reluctant to conform to the denial behaviour which was an institutional dynamic in the workplace, and would leave. This indicates a tension in remaining sensitive and aware of one's feelings amongst staff who defend themselves from such feelings. As described in Chapter 14, these behaviours may belong to the organisation. Staff may use behaviour which in another setting they would not consider;

A nurse sat alone in a side room next to a cot with an infant in it who had died the day before. She drank her coffee and ate a biscuit as she waited for the parents to enter the room.

A young woman asked to see a family at a hospice and to pay her last respects to her friend. The staff told her that no one was there at present and she was shown into the room where her dead friend lay, and left alone.

A newly bereaved mother entered the sitting room of a hospice where the radio was playing loudly. When asked to turn it down, the staff member replied that it was to cheer everyone up.

The nurse carried out her duties in linking up the feed to a gastrostomy tube, and also administering medication, but never once looked at the young adult's face, nor spoke to the young man who was awake but unable to communicate verbally.

The above are simple examples of seeming insensitivity, but are all defensive behaviours where the emotions of having to deal fully with the pain of a situation are split off (Klein 1998).

Thinking of oneself

Health professionals are trained to put the patient first, without consideration to themselves unless it is a health and safety issue. This relates to physical health and safety. What of the emotional well-being of the health professional? This is not to supplant the patient by oneself, but to understand that working with another is a two-way process. This usually means that the patient is in a passive role and the health professional is in a dominant role. How this dominance is used and interpreted by the different health professionals varies from 'doing with' the patient to 'doing for' and 'doing to' the patient.

Rehabilitation therapists including occupational therapists, physiotherapists, and speech and language therapists can be faced with real difficulties in palliative care (see Ch. 4) as training focuses upon improvement and discharge, not deterioration and dying as in the palliative care paradigm. Uncertainty, conflict and tension (Bye 1998) arise from working with people who have palliative care needs. This can be further aggravated for the therapist when palliative care is one approach needed amongst others in the space of a day. When a patient dies, a member of staff can be left with the feelings of frustration of the person in not having achieved or completed all that had been wished. It can also be the member of staff who feels the frustration of not having done something for the patient.

> Therapist: 'I was so close to arranging for Mrs White to go home. She wanted to die at home and she didn't, she died on the ward. I feel I let her down.'

There may be work left undone. This aspect of not having achieved all that was intended over time can affect one's professional confidence. This is often combined with the feelings of grief and loss, which are also felt. Although this grief is not to the same degree and depth as it would be for a loved one or close relative, the impact of a patient dying is felt acutely, but an organisation may not acknowledge staff feelings, nor encourage them to be discussed or shown in the workplace. Perhaps this is a defensive function (Zagier-Roberts 2002, p. 114) due to an anxiety on the part of the management that such feelings may not be contained, and can threaten to overwhelm the organisation and its functional capacity. This can leave a health professional feeling unsupported and uncertain. If there are other aspects of uncertainty affecting professional identity and task then deskilling can occur.

> Occupational therapist at a children's hospice: 'It took me some time to realise that making beds, running baths, and occasionally cleaning a child's room was positively contributing to the tasks of the team as a whole, but didn't limit nor define my own core skills.'

Personal quiz

This is an informal self-test, devised by the author, to provide an idea of how one feels in work, and about one's own work. It may help identify when fatigue, feelings of deskilling, and frustration are occurring.

Score between 0–5 for each question (unless specified). For example, the first question can be scored 0 if there is no sense of fulfilment at all, and 5 for the maximum level of fulfilment.

For the negatively scored examples, e.g. Question 8 'At times I feel unsure about what I am doing', if answering 'extremely unsure' then this is minus 5. If the answer is 'very sure of what I am doing', then mark yourself as 0. There are gradations in between 0–5 but this mark is written down as a minus and deducted from the total score.

Read each statement quickly and score yourself:

1. I feel fulfilled in my work.
2. I know I make a difference.
3. Referrals/requests made to me are appropriate.
4. My multi-professional team colleagues are aware of my skills and role.
5. I have good support for my role as .... (enter discipline).
6. I get good support as a member of the team on a personal level.
7. I enjoy my work.
8. At times I feel unsure about what I am doing (score minus 0–5).
9. I receive praise and positive feedback.

185

10. My job appraisals are helpful and my manager is knowledgeable of my role, skills and contribution.

11. I achieve my aims.

12. My level of frustration at work is ..... (score minus 0–5).

13. I find it harder to be motivated (score minus 0–5).

14. I am feeling tired – physically and emotionally (score minus 0–5).

Add up the scores, remembering to deduct the minus scores for questions 8, 12, 13, and 14.

The total score achieved when feeling fulfilled, confident and valued in one's work is 50.

The score is an informal indicator of feelings about one's work. It should be recognised that there are good days and bad days in palliative care, as there are good weeks and bad weeks. Good and bad times are usually determined by recognition of work done, and of staff grief. Whilst there is a lot written about bereavement when someone dies, there is little about the impact on a member of staff working with terminally ill and dying people. (See Chs 6 and 13 for further information.)

Staff grief

Palliative care settings are usually calm and gentle places, not associated with fast, active, time-pressured settings where deadlines have to be met, and there is no palpable sense of urgency.

> 'I thought it would be quite stressful here, but there is so much more time to do things than on the ward,' commented a student nurse on starting a placement at a hospice.

Stress in palliative care presents quite differently. It can be a residual low-level stress of knowing that all of the patients have a life-limiting condition. The stress increases at times when someone dies. When someone dies, there is still a lot of work to be done, in supporting the family, in looking after the body and moving the body of the deceased person. No one can be prepared for this regardless of how often it may have occurred.

> Occupational therapist at a hospice: 'A young man had died but had requested that he be buried in his favourite football strip. His parents knew this and were keen that his wish was carried out. One of the nurses, Sam, and I were free and so we agreed to do this. I felt nervous as I had last seen this young man, James, when he was alive. Sam said she had done this sort of thing before. We needed to wash and dress this young man. I had not been involved in such a task before. James was to be placed into his coffin that evening. We collected the clothes, and James' own toiletries. We put on plastic aprons and rubber gloves before we went into the room where he had lain for 4 days. Sam knocked on the door, and called his name. She said we were coming in and said my name too. We went into the cold room (kept cold for the body). We each said hallo. He was yellow and waxy looking in appearance. His body was cold to touch and he was stiff. We each spoke to him throughout the washing and drying. The water was warm. I had been keen to make sure it was neither too hot nor too cold for him. I never considered using cold water. Dressing James was difficult because he was so stiff. I

wanted to cry and struggled not to. Afterwards Sam and I cleared away and each said goodbye to James. As I was empting the water, and taking the towels to the laundry Sam was called away by another nurse to assist with medication. I washed the bowls over again before putting them into the sluice. The rest of the hospice was warm and noisy, in such contrast to the room we had been in with James. I still had the rest of the day to work, but felt physically and emotionally numb and cold. I made hot tea for Sam and myself. I was surrounded by other people talking, and music on the radio. But I felt numb and probably in a state of shock I suppose. Hot tea and a chocolate biscuit – contrasting with James who was so still and cold. Sam took hers and carried on writing in the file. I felt very sad and numb inside. It was as if everything was carrying on as normal when things were not normal at all. Sam and I exchanged a few words, acknowledging how difficult it was to move James but that he was dressed as had requested and now was ready for his coffin and funeral. I don't remember what I did for the rest of that afternoon, but I remember how fast I drove home, how much I hugged my own children when I saw them, and how I had opened wine, sitting in the warm kitchen, just crying. My husband was sympathetic and hugged me. I thought of James. I lit a candle and said some words to say goodbye as I did so. I went to work the next day but could not go to the funeral as we were short staffed, and it was already accepted that only a few staff could ever be released to attend a funeral at one time.'

Staff grief does happen, and it is a valid and stressful experience (Lenart et al 1998). It can threaten to disrupt the ongoing work with other patients who are living. Consequently, staff who are struggling with their grief may not be comforted by colleagues who are also struggling to manage their own feelings at work when the primary task is still to care for people who are living and requiring staff assistance. Whilst staff are actively involved in supporting individual family members in their grief and bereavement, that of the staff members is overshadowed by the purpose of their work of helping another. It is the key worker(s) who are most affected when a patient dies. The key worker will have built up a professional relationship with the patient – of trust, of getting to know the person and the family. It is also the key worker(s) who the family turn to and look to for support immediately after the death. It is the key workers who are affected by grief of their own which has to be delayed in order for them to carry out tasks and support the family. How long this is delayed varies.

Therapist: 'It was only when we had a remembering service for the staff and spoke of the 10 young people who had died over the last 8 weeks that I realised I had not stopped to think about them all properly. When I stopped and sat down to think about this I just cried. I felt as if I had been holding it all in myself, but couldn't let it go because I could not have done my work with the families I had been key worker for.'

There is a shared intimacy in caring for people who are dependent upon aspects of self-care such as washing and toileting, and a trust and relationship develops which is especially poignant when the patient is dying. This occurs in other situations in the health service apart from palliative care. However, whilst the tasks of bereavement and bereavement itself are widely understood as normal but painful processes, with an ensuing emotional turmoil in order for readjustment to be reached for health (Worden 1995), the impact upon staff and the daily acknowledgement in work is less understood and recognised. The unwritten code is that staff members must be able to draw upon their own strengths to get them through so that they are not overcome by their grief or that of others. It is as if staff grief is not legitimate (White 2005). All health professionals who work with dying patients are affected, and the longer the time spent with someone the more vulnerable the person (Redinbaugh et al 2003).

Grief can accumulate and can affect the ability of staff to provide care, and perform their duties (Feldstein & Gemma 1995). Grief cannot be avoided, indeed it needs to happen if staff are to care and work sensitively in palliative care. One develops a relationship with patients over time. However one's grief can compound any existing difficulties such as feelings of stress, or of being undervalued.

Recognition of one's own feelings and of grief is important. It is important to be alert to one's feelings, which is not comfortable. A small ritual can be helpful.

> Nurse: 'I have found that going home and lighting a special candle, and thinking of the person helps. Sometimes I will take half an hour, to think about the person, and say goodbye.'

Such a ritual is personal and often not understood by one's own family. Loved ones will be concerned and suggest that it might be time to leave the job and work elsewhere. Working in palliative care is still relatively new and can be viewed in different ways by one's friends and family. Such attitudes and responses can unwittingly further isolate and undermine.

> Occupational therapist: 'I remember when I was about to start work at a hospice and a friend asked me, "Why do you want to work there?" as if I had a morbid interest or something. Even another therapist who works in acute medicine asked, "When are you going to leave?" just after I had started! They didn't understand and, if anything, I felt I had to justify what I was doing at work to people outside of work as well as colleagues at work when I started.'

Compassion fatigue

Below are some comments made by staff working in different settings, which are not exclusive to working in palliative care:

'Sometimes everyone is a priority, and I go home late.'

'When it's really busy, I don't stop, and when I get home I just feel exhausted on every level.'

'I am leaving. I just can't keep giving out anymore. I think I've got compassion fatigue.'

Samuel Oliner et al (1992) wrote of the altruistic personality, identifying three main characteristics which set those who possessed it apart from others. These were:

1. a wish to help another
2. a greater sense of responsibility
3. a heightened empathy to pain.

In addition, such people act instinctively without thoughts for the self. Extreme altruism can lead to sacrifice of one's life in saving another, as witnessed in war. These three qualities are seen in people who work with the traumatised, and bereaved children and adults (Dyregrov, unpublished work, 1998). Such people have a strong impulse to help others. This links with one's motivation to work in a particular field of care, in this case palliative. Such motivations may be conscious or unconscious and linked to one's own life experience (Bennett 1991). It may be uncomfortable to consider why one chooses to work in a particular medical field. However, doing so can provide clues to one's own motivational drive and what is being sought. It can also help identify why some situations, or families can have more of an emotional effect than others.

All of these aspects require an emotional stamina and resilience for health professionals in their work. However, one is human and can become emotionally upset at times, even exhausted. It is not inevitable that everyone experiences some sort of compassion fatigue, of being tired and drained. Compassion fatigue is a sort of tiredness, which can present physically as well as emotionally. It affects people who are sensitive, caring and compassionate to others in an environment where others are in need of understanding and care. Compassion fatigue can affect the ability to care compassionately. It can lead to an emotional distancing by the member of staff when working with a child, or adult. This can take many forms: choosing not to pick up cues when someone appears 'flat'; avoiding emotionally demanding situation(s); focusing on administrative tasks, etc. It can also affect professional relationships, e.g. feeling too tired to put a point of view across, not asking colleagues if they are OK when you think they may not be, not wanting to participate or volunteer for projects, etc. All of these examples require energy. Compassion fatigue seems to be a half-way stage to burnout. It is not burnout, as there is a possible recovery from compassion fatigue. Holidays, a positive spate occurring in work, the esteem of colleagues can all contribute to a recovery. The ability to recover one's energy, drive and commitment is linked to being able to recognise when one is beginning to feel tired. However, it is not always so and compassion fatigue can continue until a person reaches burnout.

Ironically, burnout can affect effective people, who are active and energetic – usually those people who put in the extra effort in their work. Everyone has a different threshold for stress, and the key is to know one's own stress level. Freudenberger & Richelson (1980) identified burnout, defining it as a state of fatigue or frustration due to a relationship, a cause or way of life which has not produced a desired result or reward. This is linked to unrealistic or unattainable goals. Motivation and the goals associated with it are important to identify, as one may be setting oneself up for stress and frustration. Stress builds as time becomes more pressured. Trying to fit everything into the time at work begins to affect home life. As stress builds, a sense of hopelessness and helplessness (Schaie & Willis 1996) develops. This can reinforce a sense of deskilling, and loss of professional confidence. Cumulative stress has different phases which can develop over years (Annscheutz 1999) and become part of one's behaviour. Milstein et al (2002) recognise the emotional vulnerability of staff and advocate a debriefing system. This identifies five aspects; the background of the situation; how it affects thinking and feeling; identifying the troublesome or difficult elements; the behaviour or handling of these difficulties; and support to empower the person and to reach a satisfactory conclusion. The difficulty for some staff is recognising when they are emotionally tired, and on the way to exhaustion and burnout. It is important therefore to regularly reflect upon one's feelings about work. In many ways difficulties are related to finding meaning and purpose in one's own life, and being able to help others recognise these for themselves too. For many staff in palliative care there is an affirmation of the value and importance of life, which is perceived as positive and enriching.

References

Annscheutz B A 1999 The high cost of caring . . . coping with workplace stress. OACAS (Ontario Association of Children's Aid Societies) Journal 43(3):17–21

Bennett S 1991 Issues confronting occupational therapists working with terminally ill patients. British Journal of Occupational Therapy 54(1):8

Bye R 1998 When clients are dying: occupational therapists' perspectives. Occupational Therapy Journal of Research 18(1):3–24

Feldstein M A, Gemma P B 1995 Oncology nurses and chronic compounded grief. Cancer Nursing Journal 18(3):228–236

Freudenberger H, Richelson G 1980 Burnout: the high cost of high achievement. Doubleday, New York

Klein M 1998 The psycho-analysis of children. Karnac, London

Lenart S B, Bauer C G, Brighton D D et al 1998 Grief support for nursing staff in the ICU. Journal for Nurses in Staff Development 14(6):293–296

Mawson C 2002 Containing anxiety in work with damaged children. In: Obholzer A, Zagier-Roberts V (eds) The unconscious at work. Brunner-Routledge, London

Menzies I E P 1960 Social systems as a defence against anxiety: an empirical study of the nursing service of a general hospital. In: Trist E, Murray H (eds) The social engagement of social science. Vol. 1: The socio-psychological perspective. Free Association, London

Milstein J M, Gerstenberger A E, Barton S 2002 Healing the caregiver. Journal of Alternative and Complementary Medicine 8(6):917–920

Oliner S, Oliner P, Baron L et al 1992 Embracing the other: philosophical, psychological and historical perspectives on altruism. New York Press, New York

Redinbaugh E M, Sullivan A M, Block S D et al 2003 Doctors' emotional reactions to recent death of a patient: cross sectional study of hospital doctors. British Medical Journal 327:185. Online. Available: www.bmj.bmjjournals.com/cgi/content/full/327/7408/ 2 Nov 2006

Schaie W K, Willis S L 1996 Adult development and ageing. HarperCollins, New York, pp 231–232

Speck P 2002 Working with dying people. In: Obholzer A, Zagier-Roberts V (eds) The unconscious at work. Brunner-Routledge, London

White K 2005 Statewide trek: a journey for health workers going through grief loss. Paper presented at National Rural Health Conference March 10–13 Alice Springs, Australia. Online. Available: www.ruralhealth.org.au

Worden J 1995 Grief counselling and grief therapy. Routledge, London

Zagier-Roberts V (2002) The self-assigned impossible task. In: Obholzer A, Zagier-Roberts V (eds) The unconscious at work. Brunner-Routledge, London

Suggested further reading

Burnout Inventory. Online. Available: www.lessons4living.com/burnout_inventory2htm 31 Oct 2006

Igodan O C, Newcomb L H 1986 Are you experiencing burnout? Journal of Extension 24(1). Online. Available: www.joe.org/joe/1986spring/a l.html 30 Oct 2006

Palliative Care Council for South Australia 2006 Caring for yourself in the face of compassion fatigue. Online. Available: http://www.pallcare.asn.au 3 Nov 2006

If –

I

If you can keep your head when all about you
Are losing theirs and blaming it on you,
If you can trust yourself when all men doubt you
But make allowance for their doubting too;
If you can wait and not be tired by waiting,
Or being lied about, don't deal in lies,
Or being hated, don't give way to hating,
And yet don't look too good, nor talk too wise:

II

If you can dream – and not make dreams your
   master;
If you can think – and not make thoughts your aim;
If you can meet with Triumph and Disaster
And treat those two impostors just the same;
If you can bear to hear the truth you've spoken
Twisted by knaves to make a trap for fools,
Or watch the things you gave your life to, broken,
And stoop and build 'em up with worn-out tools:

III

If you can make one heap of all your winnings
And risk it on one turn of pitch-and-toss,
And lose, and start again at your beginnings
And never breathe a word about your loss;
If you can force your heart and nerve and sinew
To serve your turn long after they are gone,
And so hold on when there is nothing in you
Except the Will which says to them: 'Hold on!'

IV

If you can talk with crowds and keep your virtue,
Or walk with Kings – nor lose the common touch,
If neither foes nor loving friends can hurt you;
If all men count with you, but none too much,
If you can fill the unforgiving minute
With sixty seconds' worth of distance run,
Yours is the Earth and everything that's in it,
And – which is more – you'll be a Man, my son!

Rudyard Kipling

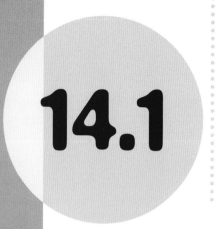

Appendix 14.1
Strategies for keeping going

Claire Tester

Sometimes working in palliative care, it can be difficult to perceive what one is doing. A psychotherapist once remarked, 'It must seem like all of your work and energy is going into a black hole when someone dies.' Although this is not a view upheld by the majority of staff, it does highlight the thought that regardless of energies and effort by different health professionals the patient cannot be made better, and the person dies. This thought may accumulate at an unconscious level and lead to a crisis of self-confidence, a feeling of deskilling, and uncertainty for an individual. Such feelings are often linked to unresolved grief when patients die. This may occur after a few months, or even years.

Some ideas for working in palliative care in a positive and healthy way are given here. There will be many other ideas, and not all of these may appear relevant to each person, but can provide a start for thinking about oneself at work and how personal aims and objectives can be identified. Ideas are separated into broad categories but are not exclusive. All of the ideas can be utilised by anyone. When vulnerable and unsure about role, it is necessary to remind oneself positively of skills and experience to date.

1. Identify the core skills of your own profession. When you are confident in your own core skills, and specialist skills, discuss them with your colleagues. Write them down and make them accessible, e.g. for those who refer to you. This ensures referrals are appropriate and informs staff who may change and may be unsure. Often such an exercise encourages others to consider their core skills, and areas of professional overlap can be safely identified.

2. Look at your own curriculum vitae (c.v.), listing your skills and experience. This c.v. may need updating as further skills and experience will have been gained.

3. Use the updated c.v. in individual supervision and job appraisal meetings with your manager. The identified core skills can be used too if the manager is unclear about the role and the contribution you can make.

4. Use a spare page at the back of your diary. Write down three headings spaced down the page of: Aims; Work in progress; and Achievements. (If you do not have a diary it is helpful to have one, even if part way through the year, as significant personal events can be recorded as they occur.)

   Aims. Thinking about your own aims in work, what is it you want to achieve at your workplace? These can be broken down into immediate, medium, and long-term goals. An example of a medium-term aim might be to introduce a revised or new assessment checklist form, or a referral sheet to inform your colleagues. It can be hard to set aims and this will take some time to consider, but without aims and a sense of direction, it can be hard to know the direction and the next step forward.

   Work in progress. This should already link in with your aims in the work you are doing and have yet to complete. It is helpful to identify what you are doing and at what stage you are at, perhaps near to completion.

Achievements. Write down what has been accomplished by you, regardless of how small or insignificant you might consider the achievement to be. This includes courses, seminars and lectures attended, and given. Another example might be the review of a risk assessment.

The reason for keeping these headings at the back of the diary is that every time something is done it can be noted down in the diary. This provides an ongoing record, and enable one to see more readily what is being accomplished.

5. As a new member of staff, when starting a new position it can be helpful to first identify what everyone else does, rather than to meet colleagues and tell them what you are going to do. It is important to listen to others first, and to discern what the function of the team is and how individual members perceive their own role. This approach can highlight gaps in the service, and the role others expect you to fill.

Occupational therapist at a hospice: 'When I spoke to different team members and found out what was happening, I could clearly see what was not happening and where I could positively contribute to the work of the team. For me initially it was positioning a child, identifying correct seating, informal assessments of a child's developmental and cognitive abilities, and using this information to tactfully identify activities and ideas for therapeutic play.'

In a new position or new service it is important to work alongside your colleagues actively – getting your hands dirty, contributing to unpleasant chores at times. Working a full day shift or over a day and evening can provide an insight into the day in the life of a patient, as well as staff. This quickly enables one to gain an insight into how the team works and the service provided. On an informal note it demonstrates a willingness to work alongside other staff members and an active interest in their work. Working relationships are helped along in this way. New members of staff can often feel on the outside of a team as they try to fathom its workings. Being new in a situation can allow you to ask basic questions about what is going on, and 'to make time and space for (one's) observations and experiences' (Obholzer 2002).

6. Be clear about what you can do in your professional role. This also means being clear about what you cannot do, what is appropriate, and when the skills of someone else are required. It is understandable, but preventable, when health professionals set themselves an impossible task, to provide the very best they can at all times (Zagier-Roberts 2002, p. 113). This creates enormous pressure for an individual, and a team collectively, leading to recriminations of others not pulling their weight, of sacrifices of time; staying late, arriving early and not claiming time back.

To consider the impossibility of being perfect and to provide consistently good-enough care, therapy, or treatment of a patient may need to be enough (Dartington 2002, Speck 2002).

7. Use opportunities appropriately to explain your role whether one-to-one, or at a team meeting. This can also be shared through case presentations or work done. It is helpful to discuss and share with all staff who may have different experiences of working with your own professional role.

A paediatric occupational therapist describes: 'It was a large meeting for a case discussion. When it came to my turn, I outlined what I had done and also what the OT role could offer to contribute to the case. The social worker who had worked with OTs in social services regarding adaptations etc. loudly accused me of making my job up as I went along. It was unnecessary and embarrassing. Although I spoke with her afterwards, it proved difficult for team members at the meeting to discuss my contribution further.'

193

8. Ensure that you are included on new staff induction programmes so that you have an opportunity to meet new staff on the team and are able to tell them what you do. This contributes to clarity for the new staff members and reinforces the work of the team and roles within the team. New staff are also provided with an opportunity to question and discuss aspects of your role which they may not do otherwise, but guess at.

9. Take yourself seriously in your work and others will follow. This is especially true of a new position or role within a team.

10. Identify other health professionals who have a similar role to you elsewhere. Contact them for professional support, peer review, and information. Such relationships can be supportive and helpful.

11. Find out about specialist groups, and professional meetings which are applicable to you, and are of interest and relevance to your work.

> Physiotherapist: 'I had not realised how much I missed the shared language until I met up with other physiotherapists. There is an automatic understanding and appreciation of the role of the physio when you meet them. I didn't have to explain myself. We shared experiences and approaches in problem solving. It was so valuable'.

12. Establish regular contact with a professional colleague you can trust and share views or concerns with, for peer review, or for supervision. Supervision may take place every 6–10 weeks and provides an opportunity for one's work to be discussed confidentially. It is not case supervision but enables aims, objectives, and achievements to be raised as well as aspects of conflict or tension which may need discussion in this neutral setting.

13. Write up any positive encounter, piece of work, therapy, approach or treatment you have been directly involved in which has been successful. This enables a review and contributes to continuing professional development (CPD), as well as encouraging the practice of writing for a journal etc.

14. Every 6 months take the opportunity to review and evaluate what you have done and where you are. This is for yourself and is not related to a manager's request. Use the three headings (see point 4 above) and record at the back of your diary as a start for your own review. At the end of each year look at your own work within a setting, even though this work setting may have changed since the last personal review. Through looking over your work it will be possible to identify any difficulties, or aspects of work you wish to develop further. This is also an opportunity to identify trends and patterns in working which are unhelpful, or helpful. For example, one therapist noted that she was receiving referrals for younger children with increasingly complex needs. This was in marked contrast to her previous referrals of mainly young adults. This was identified as a new role of young adult worker on the team, and a recognition of her own skills with developmentally delayed children. This led to an audit by the team of all referrals received.

15. A personal project which would add value to your own work and that of the team in improving service to patients, can be positive in many ways. It does not have to have a time limit, and may involve others. The idea of nurturing and developing something which is sustainable when patients are ill and dying, can be helpful and rewarding. Such a project is an adjunct to the main body of work, and may be 'picked up' and 'dropped' at different times. This may stem from identifying an area of need, or a resource.

16. Take and make opportunities for your own learning. This may be distance learning, or setting up a journal or specific seminar sessions.

17. Reflective practice is helpful, and although felt by many to be time consuming it does not have to be so. Even a 5-minute thinking time at the end of each day, specifically to think over what

has gone well, or has been difficult, is useful before going home. It can be easier to take one's work away in the mind, and to unwind it at home. However, difficulties at work often cannot be discussed at home because of confidentiality, and a reflective time before going home helps to review what has happened. Dr Atle Dyregrov maintains that writing out difficulties in a reflective piece can actively lower the tension in the body. 'It is not enough to just write about what happened; you have to write about your deepest thoughts and emotions about the event too. Then it has a therapeutic effect.'

18. To present and speak about aspects of your work enables a sharing of experiences with others, and encourages discussion. This also encourages a confidence in public speaking. Deskilling of one's own work and role can lead to a lack of confidence, when often one's own experience can be echoed by others, including deskilling.

19. When a lone practitioner, having a student on placement can provide an opportunity to double the presence of your health profession. It always involves more work but besides supporting a student, there is an opportunity to firm up and develop aspects of one's own role.

20. Value yourself as an individual because your energy levels and confidence inspire others – both patients and colleagues.

21. Coping mechanisms vary for each person when working with patients at an emotional level, but when and how can defences be dropped? Are they dropped at home, or before?

> One colleague said to me: 'I just didn't have time to think. I was working three long shifts on the go. When I got to the weekend I went to a party, I just drank so much. It was so unlike me. I just wanted to let go. You know, forget, but I didn't.'

Some recreational activities can act as defences in denying one's emotions, e.g. drinking alcohol to excess. What sort of recreational activities do we choose for ourselves? It can be difficult to make time for oneself. The importance of relaxation, of winding down is important but this becomes difficult as stress builds. Stress and emotions can accumulate, becoming knotted so that there is no identifiable start or finish that can be easily unravelled.

22. When not at work, what do you find personally uplifting? What do you enjoy doing? How often do you do these things?

23. Write down what you would like more of in your life generally? How can you get this?

24. These last two points may indicate a need to reorganise one's own life out of work. This is not easy with children or partners. It is very easy to extend a situation of giving and doing at work and to extend it at home, e.g. rushing home to meet children, to shop, to prepare a meal for another, to say nothing of washing, ironing, paying bills, etc. When do you unwind? Have you found a way? Can you identify it?

25. From time to time identify your own stress levels. The irony is that stress builds and can become overwhelming, leading to burnout and exhaustion and ill health.

26. When working as a lone practitioner, especially in a new position, and developing one's role, the amount of energy and effort put into work can lead to stress. It can also lead to an over-commitment to one's role and a sense of being indispensable, which one needs to aware of.

Organisational support

Besides individual strategies for oneself, strategies for the well-being of the staff group need to be recognised as necessary by the organisation. All individuals have their own levels of stress and ways of coping, but for those in a team, the team itself needs to be alert to the needs of its individual members (Owen 2000). Some ideas include a staff counsellor, debriefing meetings after a death, a staff group with a counsellor, remembrance services – weekly, monthly, annually. Also 'staff away' days and staff social occasions can help develop camaraderie but must include new staff. New staff can often feel on the outside of an established team.

References

Dartington A 2002 Where angels fear to tread. In: Obholzer A, Zagier-Roberts V (eds) The unconscious at work. Brunner-Routledge, London

Obholzer A 2002 Afterword. In: Obholzer A, Zagier-Roberts V (eds) The unconscious at work. Brunner-Routledge, London, p 210

Owen R 2000 Relieving stress in palliative care staff. Palliative Care Today 9(1):4–5

Speck P 2002 Working with dying people. In: Obholzer A, Zagier-Roberts V (eds) The unconscious at work. Brunner-Routledge, London

Zagier-Roberts V (2002) The self-assigned impossible task. In: Obholzer A, Zagier-Roberts V (eds) The unconscious at work. Brunner-Routledge, London

All that was left ... hope

Kathryn Boog with Claire Tester

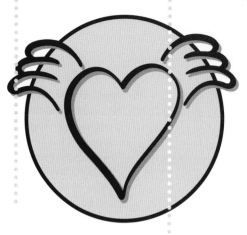

Hope is the mechanism that keeps the human race tenaciously alive, dreaming, planning, building.
Hope is not the opposite of realism ... it is the opposite of cynicism and despair.

Ardeth Whiteman

Key words

Pandora's box; meanings and values; goals; spirituality; humour; mirroring

Chapter contents

15

According to Greek myth, Pandora opened the forbidden box belonging to her wise husband Epimetheus, and unwittingly unleashed all the evils and ills into the world. They stung Pandora and she slammed the lid shut, trying to protect herself. She heard a voice calling her from inside the box, pleading to be let out, and when she opened the lid, out flew Hope, the only thing left in the box. It gently touched her wounds, healing the hurt and then flew off into the world to follow the miseries that had been unleashed.

Without hope in humanity there is despair, for without hope there is no possibility for change in improvement of a situation or circumstance. As Christine Longaker (1997) says, 'Most of us feel that living is hopeful and that death represents the loss of hope. Yet hope can be experienced on many levels, and what is hopeful while we are living is in fact the same hope we can cultivate when we are dying'.

Hope is moulded by a wide array of influences such as culture, ethnicity and life experiences, and changes over the illness journey (Jones 2005). People search for the meanings and values that have been important to them and have guided their path, and use these to influence and select new goals. They reprioritise, and these new goals may be more in tune with the spiritual element of their being (Puchalski 2002), allowing them to transcend their difficulties and by striving for, and attaining, mastery over their present circumstances, adjust to their new situation (van der Lee et al 2005), In order to achieve this, new goals must be realistic and meaningful, and because of the shifting nature of progressive and terminal disease, the goalposts need to be flexible and moveable.

It is just this possibility of potential change that is encouraging when times are difficult. Hope enables many people to live, and acts as a spur for getting through a difficult time. Hope becomes part of an individual's belief system that things may get better. It is not positive thinking, which is better defined as a therapeutic or systematic process to counter pessimism, and neither is it optimism, for hope is imbued with emotion and has feeling as well as thinking *with it*. For some, hope is in the form of wishes, dreams or prayer. Hope in dying is linked both to living and to the hope of what will happen at and after death, so it has a spiritual dimension. Hope can be shared but is personal, and should not be taken away by another as it can sustain life, even though it might be perceived as fantasy. As long as hope is not creating unsafe decisions or actions, it is generally viewed as a positive thing.

Hope in dying is sometimes disparaged by others as being false and without any basis in truth. It may be rooted in denial, which can serve a valuable purpose as a coping strategy when the odds seem overwhelming, but continued denial may be one style of false hope (Centers 2001) based on untruths, and is untenable in the longer term.

Hopelessness, on the other hand, may be due to a weariness with life (Cassidy 1991) and a feeling that control over the situation is lost (Byrne 2002) leading to demoralisation and despair (Kissane et al 2001).

It is beginning to be understood that there is a mind–body connection, that one's emotions and thinking can affect some physical changes, either positively or negatively (Seligman & Martin 1992). This is linked to positive psychology, which recognises that it is easier to be negative than positive. In this way optimism is linked to hope and confidence (Kivimaki et al 2005).

In palliative care the person can be 'turned' into a patient with all the associated passivity of the traditional role. However, by empowering people, through support and choice, assisted decision making and being actively involved, making choices in their own life and for their own life, a positive outlook is encouraged which fosters hope.

'People's emotional responses to terminal illness can determine whether they live actively and positively, maintaining a hopeful outlook, or whether they are consumed by fear of what is happening to them or have anxieties about the future' (Lugton 2002).

Individuals' belief systems, influenced by cultural, ethnic and spiritual values will significantly direct their aspirations for a successful outcome. The meanings that they make from their lives and their successes and failures will provide the background for hopes for the future. This is fully discussed in Chapter 11. Activities that respond to these individual needs are responding to the existential aspects of a person's life, making meaning and fostering hope (Lyons et al 2002).

There are differences between individuals in having hope, and a positive outlook on life and death. One's own cultural upbringing affects this, as well as a national culture. For example, in India the idea of no hope for cure is not discussed, as there is medical collusion with the families to pursue active treatments even at the cost of financial ruin (Maddocks 2003).

Hope is part of everyday life and carries meaning and a real wish for realised action. It is found in everyone's everyday conversation:

'I hope the bus is on time.'
'I hope I can get home before it gets dark.'

Hope for the patient

In palliative care hope can be based on a vision of what can still be achieved rather than dwelling on what is no longer possible (Hockley 1993). Supporting hope means looking at the wider picture and directing patients in the reframing of their goals and their dreams, based on the changing focus of their lives now that those lives have changed irrevocably and forever.

Hope stretches into the future – for some it is a little way ahead:

'I hope I can eat the lunch today, as it was difficult to swallow yesterday.'
'I hope my daughter visits today.'
'My Dad hopes they will find a cure for his cancer soon.'
'I hope to see my son's wedding next month.'
'I hope to meet my wife in heaven.'
'I hope my daughter will meet her Gran in heaven and they can look after each other.'

whilst for others, it travels to a more distant future:

'I want to make my daughter's party dress so that I can still be a part of her birthday.'
'She will receive all the birthday cards I've made for her and she'll know how much I wanted to be there.'
'I'll make the little knick-knacks for his room and he'll remember me when he sees them.'
'I've made the favours for the wedding. That way I'll be there in their thoughts.'

Continuity and hope for the future is promoted by families' adherence to their traditions even after the death of the person who was responsible for these (Syren et al 2006).

Generativity may also be assured in the form of legacy and leaving gifts, a major contributor to feelings of hope. These may be for loved ones, or may take the form of items made for sale in the hospice shop, where patients feel that they are giving something back. They can also be donations such as CD players, books, paintings, etc. for future patients to benefit from.

Many people still hope to achieve things before they die, and learning a new activity such as painting or using the computer, or seeing children married or grandchildren born, offers scope for this to be addressed. Learning new skills can counteract feelings of helplessness, hopelessness and uselessness (Lyons et al 2002), whilst looking forward to landmark events is an aim to work towards, a goal that just might be achievable, and careful and sensitive adaptation of activities and readjustment of goals in order that an acceptable version is still possible, will ensure continued hope in the face of deteriorating abilities.

199

Mary was determined to be present at her daughter's wedding. She went shopping with one of the staff to buy her outfit and it hung by her bed for everyone to admire. When it became apparent that she would not be able to attend the ceremony, Mary made a beautiful card that was to be read out at the reception. It was decorated with pictures of red peonies, the same as her dress, and in it she said all of the things she would have wanted to tell her daughter on her wedding day. She said she knew that she had done her best. Mary died 2 days before the wedding, but her daughter said that having the card made her feel her mother was there. This was what Mary had wanted.

'Quality of life is not simply about pain control and keeping people comfortable – it is about enhancing the ability to perform an activity important to the person and family system . . . creating opportunities to live fully and productively until death.'

(Pizzi 1984)

The use of humour in palliative care to engender hope was described in a recent study (Adamle & Ludwick 2005) where it was found to be a useful coping mechanism in dealing with stress and helping patients to regain and maintain a sense of perspective on their situation. It seems totally incongruous with the concept of death and dying and yet allows for the maintenance of a normality, control of a situation, makes social interaction easier, and can help with relaxation and the relief of stress (Payne 2000). Humour is one way that patients share experiences with others in similar circumstances. Participation in group activities, whether these are creative activities, leisure activities or casual conversations, allows people to feel that they are not alone and stimulates encouragement and hope amongst the members of leisure groups (Amarshi et al 2006).

Hope for the professional

How do staff remain positive and hopeful? Various studies have attempted to reveal what it is that makes people want to work with the dying, when the general assumption is that it is a depressing and hopeless situation. In palliative care, patients want more than support and befriending – they want emotional and psychological support to be central, and balancing these with the professional's own needs as a human being can be a taxing, but necessary task in order to avoid burnout and 'stay sane'. Deciding whether or not to accept the patient's cues and open Pandora's box is a further challenge for consideration – and if the box is opened, how to deal with the consequences. This has been discussed in Chapter 7.

The personal narrative of the health professional also influences effective practice. Not only will previous life experiences influence our attitudes towards death and working with the dying (Prochnau et al 2003, Thibeult 1997), but issues for the patient may mirror personal concerns, triggering the use of avoidance tactics, such as hiding behind activities of daily living, in the struggle to deal with the emotional demands of working with the dying alongside the practical aspects of lifestyle management.

Being with the terminally ill may make people review their own thoughts on death and can arouse primitive instincts and reactions where, 'We may avoid people who are dying because on a subconscious level of magical thinking we worry that death is somehow contagious. We shouldn't worry – we're already infected! We are all HMG positive (the human mortality gene). No-one is getting out of this one alive' (Byock 2004).

The emotional toll on the professional can be overwhelming, like the evils in Pandora's box, and so caring for oneself must be a major consideration and is dealt with at length in Chapters 13 and 14. In everyday practice then, how is it possible to identify hope?

Positive outcomes stimulate hope and involve patients' trust in the professional, and the sharing of private thoughts (Rahman 2000). Witnessing the personal growth of patients and those around them, and the use of humour in the development of a sense of vitality in palliative care have been seen to enhance meaning of the experience of working in this area (Webster & Kristjanson 2002). The use of black humour amongst colleagues has been identified as a coping strategy in challenging situations, in an effort to put things into perspective and 'lift' a particular situation (Prochnau et al 2003).

Hope is encountered in many different ways and can be found in attention to the smallest detail or in the need to complete a much wider and complex set of goals, and in all of the variations in between. In order to do this, the professional has to be flexible, adaptable, resourceful and creative, but cannot be all things to all men. The focus of practice must be on the patient's needs, but without consciously being aware of it, professionals begin to look at life differently, to look for meaning in both their professional and personal lives, to reframe priorities, and to seek many of the goals that they identify in their patients. By creating and developing their own values, these professionals imbue hope not only in their patients, but also in themselves.

Presenting case studies or 'narratives of client work' (Bond 2002) is a way of sharing ideas and outcomes with colleagues, and they may be able to link the story with a similar situation in their own practice, encouraging hope in a situation that they felt was not as positive as it may have been, and in this way helping them to reach closure. 'Professional closure is accomplished through objectively viewing the role the OT has in maximising the patient's quality of life' (AOTA 1986).

Mirroring

Many of the issues that arise for patients are mirrored in the professional's experiences when working with the dying. The following is an adaptation of a presentation given by the authors at the College of Occupational Therapists' annual conference in Eastbourne in July 2004, and provides an example of this theory.

Feelings about life expectancy

Mrs A: The doctor told me I don't have long to live. A poor prognosis, he said. I feel so despondent, so frightened and so helpless. What's the point of trying to do anything when I'm dying? I can't even hold a spoon properly or read a book. The nurses are doing everything for me now I'm at the hospice. I feel so useless. All washed up.

Therapist: Mrs A has such a poor prognosis and is very frail. She doesn't have much time so how can we talk about rehabilitation and learning skills to help her to cope? What can I offer? Some adapted cutlery might help, but that seems inadequate somehow. I need to find out what really matters to her – and how she's feeling.

Patient not getting better and deteriorating

Mrs A: I realise now that I'm only going to get worse. The medication for my pain is making me sleepy and so constipated. I thought I couldn't do anything for myself but yesterday they gave me some new cutlery and I could feed myself. Brian (my husband) came in and we had lunch together, in the conservatory on our own. It made such a difference to do something normal together. I still want to do things as a couple – I want him to have good memories. He won't talk about my illness. I think he's pretending it's not happening.

Therapist: Mrs A is losing skills and I have to constantly reassess her needs – almost daily now. I have been helping her with positioning to enable her to sit up, and using guided imagery and relaxation to help her cope with pain and rising panic. Mrs A has told me about her worries for her son – she is sad that she's been out of contact with him for years, and about her husband's denial of the situation. She finds it so difficult to talk to him about what's on her mind. And there's her daughter too – and her grandchildren – she is worried they won't remember her, and the good times they had.

Relationships

Mrs A: As I can't do much for myself now, I've had time to think seriously about the things that really mean a lot to me – the people I love, the people I've hurt, all the things I've done, and things I need to sort out and try to mend. What have I done with my time? How will my family and friends remember me? There are things I want to say and wish I'd said but I don't know how to do it all. Is it too late?

Therapist: Talking to Mrs A about her family has been very emotional for her. She's very distressed about her son. The card we made together with the message she wanted him to have has reached him though, and he telephoned. It's the first time she's heard from him in 14 years! She was so pleased and seemed so relieved that she said her physical pain has become more manageable. She wants to join the creative activity group – to make gifts for her family and friends. She feels she would like to thank people for caring and supporting her, and for their kindness. Working with people like Mrs A makes me reassess my own values and my own relationships, and to think about what really matters to me.

Coping mechanisms

Mrs A: My mum always said, 'Keep your head down and get on with it.' If I don't, I might break down and just sob and sob. I can't do that. What will they all think of me? That I can't cope? That would just be the last straw. So I just keep talking about my breathlessness and my pain and they won't ask me why Brian has stopped visiting me, and why my daughter doesn't bring the children in, or my friends don't phone. At the end of the relaxation session yesterday I suddenly felt so alone. The therapist spent time talking with me and really listened to what I had to say.

Therapist: I thought that if I kept to practical issues, then I wouldn't get upset so easily. I must remember to keep a professional distance – that's what I was taught. But we all have feelings, and Mrs A was so upset yesterday. As for me – I have a huge case load to manage . . . and Mr Smith died yesterday. He reminded me so much of my Uncle Jim – he died last year. Time is precious for my patients, and it's precious for me too, trying to fit everything in. I've still got all the admin to do before I go home – it's becoming more and more difficult to balance the paperwork and the clinical side of things. Tonight we'll be having a takeaway and a bottle of wine – I need some 'me' time!

Keeping going

Mrs A: Sometimes I think, 'Why am I still here?' All the treatment is making me feel so sick. I just wish it would all end. Then I think about all the things I need to get done first – just little things, but they take so much energy. Like making my son's birthday card, and telling my grandchildren how much I love them. I'm making a little memory box and filling it with photos and things and writing little stories about the things we've done together. Then they will always have a part of me. The therapist has been helping me with this. I feel as if my thoughts and memories still count and I feel respected for just being me – that makes me feel good. I'm so tired but somehow I seem to be able to find the energy to do these things. It's helped me to see that I've done my best and tried to make amends. Time is short, but very precious now.

Therapist: This new job is really challenging and it doesn't help when the other staff don't understand my role. The last therapist left though burnout, she was exhausted and ill. I am determined that that won't happen to me. I'm using reflective writing and every month or so I see a colleague for supervision. I can talk over problems and difficulties from work and my personal life. It makes such a difference to be able to let off steam. It helps me to put things into perspective. When patients are helped to achieve a goal, no matter how small, I can see that I have made a difference. Families and friends might be moved by the message in the card that the patient has made for them, or by reflections in a memory album. A memory box or final gifts will spark bittersweet memories in the recipient and help the patient to feel that they will be remembered. Reaching an estranged relative or friend and saying the things that still *need to be said all make a difference to the dying person and how they feel at the end of their life. Yes, knowing that I have been able to play a part, to help patients to do the things that they feel they need to do is what I've found most reassuring and encouraging.*

Finding meaning and purpose in life and death

Mrs A: As I die, I've been helped to think about my life and what's been important to me. I can see things from a different perspective. I want to be remembered, to feel that I've left my mark, and the staff have helped me with that and been very supportive. I have left a letter for my husband of the things I couldn't say and he can't bear to hear. I've left a memory album for my daughter and my son, and things for the grandchildren and my friends. The grandchildren won't remember me much – they're too small, but they will know who I was and how much I loved them. I have planned my funeral, and left instructions to make things easier for Brian and the family. I have been helped to look back over my life and to remember the good times. I don't feel frightened about dying. I feel ready.

Therapist: I am really pleased that I could help Mrs A to find the things that had meaning for her. She made things to be remembered by and I'll remember her and the work we did together. She thanked me before she died – and I thanked her for sharing herself with me. Working with Mrs A has made me think about what matters in my life and to reassess my priorities. Her husband spoke to me and said that although his wife hadn't been cured, they both felt that her time at the hospice and her therapy had been a healing experience.

When patients share something of themselves – their hopes and dreams as well as their failures and disappointments – health professionals realise what a privileged position they are in. Understanding the patient's story enables these professionals to foster hope in the individual through empowerment and the return of control, helping people make that transition from helplessness to hopefulness at this time of crisis, by offering opportunities for personal and emotional growth.

Seeing the difference that can be made to their patients' quality of life is when health professionals can find meaning and purpose in what *they* do, valuing skills and finding professional fulfilment and hope.

The authors' hope in this book is for improved understanding of the needs of people requiring palliative care and to provide health professionals and others interacting with people with life-limiting disease with the tools to respond to those needs.

References

Adamle K N, Ludwick R 2005 Humor in hospice care: who, where and how much? American Journal of Hospice and Palliative Medicine 22(4):287–290

Amarshi F, Artero L, Reid D 2006 Exploring social and leisure participation among stroke survivors: Part two. International Journal of Therapy and Rehabilitation 13(5):199–207

American Occupational Therapy Association (AOTA) 1986 Occupational therapy and hospice (position paper). American Journal of Occupational Therapy 40(12):839–840

Bond T 2002 Naked narrative: real research? Counselling and Psychotherapy Research 2(2):133–138

Byock I 2004 The four things that matter most. Free Press, New York, p 151

Byrne M 2002 Spirituality in palliative care: what language do we need? International Journal of Palliative Nursing 8(2):67–73

Cassidy S 1991 Terminal care. In: Watson M (ed) Cancer patient care: psychosocial treatment methods. BPS Books, Cambridge

Centers L C 2001 Beyond denial and despair: ALS and our heroic potential for hope. Journal of Palliative Care 17(4):259–264

Hockley J 1993 Rehabilitation in palliative care – are we asking the impossible? Palliative Medicine 7(1):9–15

Jones A C 2005 The role of hope in serious illness and dying. European Journal of Palliative Care 12(1):28–31

Kissane D W, Clarke D M, Street A F 2001 Demoralisation syndrome – a relevant psychiatric diagnosis for palliative care. Journal of Palliative Care 17(1):12–21

Kivimaki M, Vahtera J, Elovainio M et al 2005 Optimism and pessimism as predictors of change in health after death or onset of severe illness in family. Health Psychology 24(4):413–421

Longaker C 1997 Facing death and finding hope – a guide to spiritual care of the dying. Arrow, London, p 25

Lugton J 2002 Communicating with dying people and their relatives. Radcliffe Medical Press, Oxford

Lyons M, Orozovic N, Davis J et al 2002 Doing–being–becoming: occupational experiences of persons with life-threatening illness. American Journal of Occupational Therapy 56(3):285–295

Maddocks I 2003 Palliative care education in the developing countries. In: Rajagopal M R, Mazza D, Lipman AG (eds) Pain and palliative care in the developing world and marginalized populations: a global challenge. Haworth Press, USA, pp 211–222

Payne R A 2000 Relaxation techniques. A practical handbook for the healthcare professional. Churchill Livingstone, London

Pizzi M A 1984 Occupational therapy in hospice care. American Journal of Occupational Therapy 38(4):252–257

Prochnau C, Liu L, Bowman J 2003 Personal–professional connections in palliative care occupational therapy. American Journal of Occupational Therapy 57(2):196–204

Puchalski C M 2002 Spirituality and end-of-life care: a time for listening and caring. Journal of Palliative Medicine 5(2):289–294

Rahman H 2000 Journey of providing care in hospice: perspectives of occupational therapists. Qualitative Health Research 10(6):806–818

Seligman M, Martin E P 1992 Helplessness: on depression, development, and death. WH Freeman, New York

Syren S M, Saveman B I, Benzein E G 2006 Being a family in the midst of living and dying. Journal of Palliative Care 22(1):26–32

Thibeult R 1997 A funeral for my father's mind: a therapist's attempt at grieving. Canadian Journal of Occupational Therapy 64(3):107–114

van der Lee M L, Swarte N B, Van der Bom J G et al 2005 Positive feelings among terminally ill cancer patients. European Journal of Cancer Care 15:51–55

Webster J, Kristjanson L J 2002 'But isn't it depressing?' The vitality of palliative care. Journal of Palliative Care 18(1):15–24

Index